FIRST AID FOR YOUR MENOPAUSE EMOTIONS

FIRST AID

FOR YOUR MENOPAUSE EMOTIONS

by Patricia M. Ryan

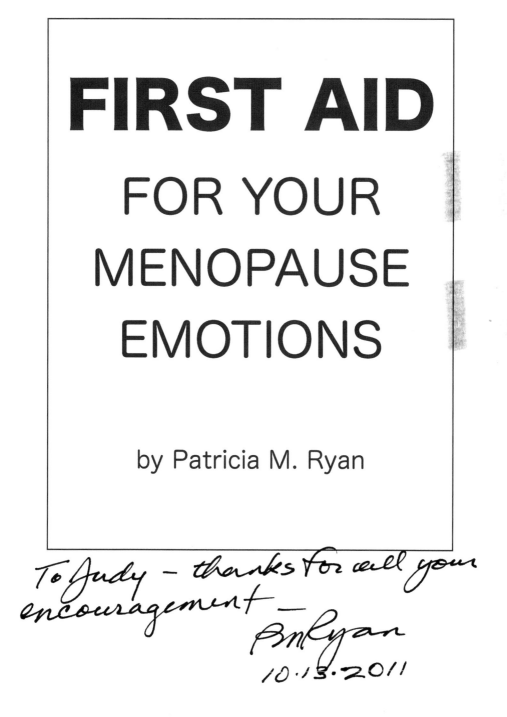

To Judy – thanks for all your
encouragement –
PMRyan
10·13·2011

Dedication

This book is dedicated to all my women friends and especially to Pam and Melissa, who helped me to conceive and write it

Life is so very much bigger than any of us

CONTENTS

Worksheets 140

All of a sudden

Once you begin to experience menopause, even sporadically, your body, mind, emotions and spirit start doing things they've never done before. Some days it's hard to keep up, especially at first when all these sensations are new and unpredictable. Observing how you feel, recording it, and writing about it can help you cope with all these changes, and not let them overwhelm you. Or at least, not so much. Would you like to have some insight into the feelings you're having ? Would you like to have ways to deal with your emotions when they seem to take over your interactions with others? Would you like to understand those days you lose to depressions that come and go of their own accord? Would you like to be able to cool down and think clearly when everything around you is driving you to distraction?

If you're experiencing symptoms of menopause, you should congratulate yourself—you are a *survivor*. You've gone over enough hurdles to qualify for the Olympics. You have survived zits, periods, school, perhaps marriage, parenthood, in−laws, and/or many years of jobs, bosses, and personnel reviews. Whether you've had children or not, you will in the foreseeable future reach a point where only a miracle could make you pregnant. You'll say goodbye to your youth, your skin tone, some part of your ambitions, your old hopes and dreams, possibly your hair, and getting carded. But guess what? You'll also be bidding a fond farewell to excruciating mammogram pain, and you'll be able to walk down the Feminine Hygiene aisle in your market and *not have to buy anything*. No more blood-stained clothes and bed linens, no sudden scary wetness at the most inconvenient times and places. If that alone isn't worth the price of admission to your adulthood, I don't know what is!

If you're not used to spending time thinking about your inner life, this book may help you get comfortable thinking—or writing—about your physical, emotional, mental and spiritual sensations, thoughts and feelings. If you're already a journaler, it will give you a tool for organizing your observations. The point of organizing it all is to help you be able to remember all your strengths and wisdom (on those days you don't think you have any), and to help you find patterns in your thoughts, your feelings, your emotional states. Menopause is going to be with you for a long time. Getting to know it early will help you find ways to cope with its events. Writing down things that are puzzling or bothering you can help put you into a more objective frame of mind, where ideas and understanding will come to you more readily.

I can think of two ways to use a menopause journal. The first would be to use it just when you've had a bad day— when you or the world or the day just didn't make sense, or when something so painful, so upsetting or unusual happened that you want a record of it. Some days you simply need to vent, and writing about how you feel and what you can't stop thinking about can really help. The second way would be to record how you feel every day for a month, or until you don't feel the need to do it any more. Maybe you've already noticed reoccurring ways of feeling, and you're trying to figure out why that might be happening. If you've never kept any kind of a journal, making your own Menopause Journal Worksheet (see Worksheet #1) can help you think of things to write about. Any feeling on it that you recognize, for instance, might spin off into thoughts about other happenings that you feel comfortable expressing. That in turn can help you to think of your daily life—and menopause—in new ways.

This book is not about hormones or hormone replacement. This book is about the everyday typical feelings of menopause that may be your steady companions for years, as your body gradually lets go of its ability to become pregnant and give birth. This is normal and natural, and for most women in their late forties or older, a sensible change. You probably have more interesting things to do than figure out how to get back inside your house after your two year old locks you out.

This book is not intended as a medical book, or to come between you and your doctor in any way. If you talk about menopause with your doctor, you should be able to ask any questions you have about it, and talk about anything that's bothering you. There are a lot of changes going on in your body and you have every right to understand them fully. The great news is that there are millions and millions of other women all around the world sharing this experience with you right now, and many of them have written comprehensive and informative books and articles about it, in print and online, and you have access to all that. They can help you sort out your experiences and decide if you want to do something about any of them.

However, that being said, I'm going to offer you two suggestions: If you haven't done so already, get your cholesterol checked, and get your thyroid checked. If they're normal, keep the records as a baseline for later.

There are many great self-help books for women, and I've read and benefited from many of them. What I hope to do with this book is encourage you to nurture yourself, no matter what kind of day you're having, no matter how you feel about any aspect of your life. This book is for all those things that frustrate you, embarrass you, confuse and exasperate you, while you feel as though your body is falling apart, you're losing your mind, and your life is going down the toilet.

If you are experiencing symptoms of menopause, you should congratulate yourself—you are a *survivor*.

Let's look at the whole picture

Throughout the decades of your thirties and forties, your life is filled with hard work, frustration, obstacles and achievements. Whether you're raising a family, working for someone else or in your own business, this is when you encounter life at its fullest. You have great tasks—and sometimes, great rewards. You learn to juggle time and demands, deal with disappointments and set your own goals.

For the most part, you're the last person you think about taking care of now; there are others who need your skills and talents and help. You're the one who figures out how to keep things running, keep everyone on schedule, solve the little problems and the big ones. How did you learn to do all this stuff? The hard way.

Then some time after your fortieth or fiftieth birthday, you wake up one morning and break a nail, and everything falls apart, nobody loves you, the world is one giant catastrophe just moments away from auto–igniting, and your whole life has lost its meaning. What happened to make that change? Did the magnetic poles shift, or the Earth come out of its orbit? No, all that happened is, your hormone levels shifted.

Sure, if you look back you can remember all those times before your period started when things were not quite right, you weren't your usual self and it was a monumental struggle to get through the day. But now here's that same situation, only tenfold. You may be going through your day feeling perfectly normal when suddenly someone says just the wrong thing and your eyes glaze over, you double in height, turn green and bite him in two. And then—you're fine again. Back to normal. Or you find yourself falling asleep at 8pm, and waking up at 3am, unable to get back to sleep. Or you go into a funk that lasts for days and drags you down into an emotional sinkhole before it goes away as quickly and mysteriously as it came.

For many women, the first symptoms of perimenopause are physical—night sweats, stuttering periods —and they can come on gradually for years before any other changes appear. The biggest problem during this early phase can be simply getting enough sleep. Later on when the emotional, mental and spiritual changes kick in, there's no part of your life that won't be affected in some way. Your periods may even start coming closer together. What, once a month isn't often enough?

What can you do to help yourself deal with all this change? How do you make sense of this? The same way you learned to make sense of everything else life has dropped you into for the last forty-something years—by observing all the things that happen, identifying how each problem affects you, and then trying different approaches till you find one that works for you.

For the ways we are affected, let's use a fairly common model of humanity. We can look at ourselves as four-fold beings: physical, mental, emotional, and spiritual. Just so we understand each other, here are some examples:

• Physical problems – headaches, gastric discomfort, tiredness, muscle pain.

• Mental problems – forgetfulness, lack of focus, distraction.

• Emotional problems – anger, resentment, self-pity, feeling alone or isolated.

• Spiritual problems – feeling disconnected, unworthy, with no purpose to your life.

If you're not feeling well physically, you won't be able to focus or concentrate, you're not going to feel spiritually connected to much of anything, and your emotions will become your first recourse when something unforeseen happens. In case you hadn't thought about this, emotions usually do not make the best recourse.

If your mind is not up to speed today, you're probably going to have to use all your energy to make up for that. If you can possibly hide in a cave and read a book or watch movies, that might be the easiest way to get through the day. However, if you have responsibilities, you'll have to put off everything you don't need to deal with, just to handle the essentials.

There is one bright spot here. Since you know without a doubt that you're not going to be able to get through the day on your own, it's easier to remember that you're in a community. Humble down and appreciate the fact that the universe can support you, that small favors and friendly gestures will appear when you really, truly need a hand. This is your spiritual connection showing up.

If you're stuck in your emotions, it's going to take all your physical strength, all your will, and all your spiritual fortitude to do anything good for yourself. Nothing is going to make sense, because emotions don't understand sense. You don't feel good enough about your body to take care of it, and the only thing you feel connected to is how many things seem wrong in your life. What you need is a good laugh, or a good cry, or both.

If your spiritual nature seems to be on another planet, if you're not feeling the joy of living today, relax. Relax, relax, relax. The odds are that you're distracted by something going on inside you right now, or some emergency in your life. The truth about your spiritual life is that it's always there, even those times you can't feel it. Focus on the things on your plate for today. Put yourself completely into them; give your heart to them. That's all you have to do. That is in fact a deep spiritual exercise, and will help reconnect you to the meaning in your life.

How can you suddenly be so vulnerable, you who were a master of living just a few months ago? Remember that ticking time clock inside you, the one that started when you hit puberty? It's striking a new hour for you. You're going to find out what you're really made of, what your real strengths are, what you're truly capable of.

You've lived long enough and through enough experiences that along with the wrinkles and stretch marks, you possess a breadth and depth of wisdom and understanding that you probably underestimate. And now suddenly, if you have never had to before, you have to pay attention to *your* feelings, to *your* needs. You have to start taking care of yourself mentally and emotionally, the same way you've been taking care of the other people in your life—your spouse, your kids, your friends, your boss and coworkers.

You have new priorities.

PRIORITY ONE: YOUR BODY

When you have a physical problem suddenly appear, how important is anything else? Imagine whacking your funny bone, stubbing your toe, serious gas pain, toothache, headache...the list is a long one. Everything else pretty much takes a back seat—doesn't it?—till you get that physical symptom taken care of in some way. Physical pain or, depending on where it is, even mild discomfort, is a major distraction from everything else you would normally be taking care of.

And even if this particular problem has happened often enough that you've learned to function through or around it, it still takes away from your focus, your concentration, and certainly your level of enjoyment. It takes energy you could be using in some more beneficial and satisfying way. My point here is that if you have a physical problem, you need to take care of it now, to make it your highest priority. Why? Because it may be a major factor in the other distressing things that are happening to you.

Your physical body isn't all there is to you, it's just a part, but it *is* the foundation that the rest of you relies upon. And at your age, it's changing. It's moving on from having been the body of a woman who can bear children while changing a tire with one hand and making a pie with the other. Or doing crosswords till after midnight and waking up at 5am to jog with hand weights for an hour before you go work an 8 or 10 or 12 hour day.

Your body is, so to speak, not so interested in doing that any more. What appeals to it now is sitting a while longer over breakfast while you read every last line of the newspaper. It would just as soon park you in a chair outside in your garden as go pull the weeds you can see from 50 feet away. It would rather watch your neighbors pack up their car for a camping trip than go wipe the crumbs off the toaster for the 9,125th time, let alone get your camping equipment together. You've been there, done that, still remember every bit, and your body knows it.

It's a sad thing about your aging body that now if you want to maintain any level of fitness or flexibility, you bloody well have to work at it. You have to make yourself do things to stay fit and flexible. Now when you really need that energy of a four year-old because there are so many wonderful and fascinating things you could go do or explore, it's gone! You don't have it any more! How much does that suck? Plenty. And if it's been a while since you did anything physical, not only are you going to have to work at it, you're going to have to be careful that you don't hurt yourself.

Some days it'll feel as though everything in your body is telling you to give up, sit down, stop working, you're just...too...tired. While you weren't looking, you suddenly went from 45 years old, to 65. When I was in my late twenties I used to do wind-sprints up alleys and think of becoming a fireman. Now I have 3 pairs of reading glasses in different places around the house so I never have to get out of my chair to go get one. Sigh.

Making yourself do something that used to come naturally doesn't just mean it's going to be tougher physically. Now you have to rearrange your life to make time to take care of yourself. Send your children off to work and get a babysitter for your husband. You have to push others out of the top spot. Many women have no idea how to put their needs first, even for one hour a week. You used to get plenty of exercise caring for others, and that was certainly okay with them. Now you have to say "Sorry, I have to take this hour when you want me to ride to the car dealer with you so I can take a nap to make up for the sleep I lost last night. No, it's not your fault I woke up, but I still need to disrupt your routine in order to make myself feel human." Or, "I don't want to make you bacon and eggs and pancakes anymore because I really want to lose ten pounds and lately I've been tasting the fat from the sausage for hours after I eat it, and the pancakes make me fart because for some unknown reason I can't digest starches any more."

Your first clue that you're approaching menopause may be waking up sweating in the middle of the night and not being able to get back to sleep. Night sweats, they call it. Personally, I don't care if I sweat a puddle, as long as I stay asleep. But if I'm lying awake at 3 am, someone is going to have to pay for that the next day. Not getting enough sleep won't just make *you* miserable, it can make everyone who interacts with you miserable.

Suddenly your energy is gone, and you can't seem to catch up on your sleep, no matter what. You're working, or are constantly interrupted during the day, so the chances of you getting to take a nap are slim to none, and Slim went off to the rodeo. You spend part or all of your day in a daze, unable to catch up with what's going on around you. You can't respond well to people because part of you might as well be shut down. Your mind doesn't work as well as you need it to, you say things even you don't understand, and your temper is about as short as a broken tampon string. Reasonable? Rational? Not so much. You struggle to get through the day, keep your mouth shut as much as possible, and try to remember all the things you were supposed to do.

The First Law Of Menopause: Catch up on your sleep.

If you have to sleep through the weekends, if you have to go to bed at 7pm, if you have to go sleep in your car, take naps at lunch, fall asleep at other people's parties—whatever you have to do—you simply *must* find a way to catch up on your sleep. Period. Nothing else will work if you don't get enough sleep.

PRIORITY TWO: YOUR EMOTIONS

Menopause may be the first time since you were a teenager, or since you gave birth, that you suddenly become an emotional being again. You cry, you're angry, and your feelings are hurt. Things that you used to take in stride make you go ballistic. A friend who said he'd call you doesn't, and now that one phone call is the most important thing in the world. Nothing else in your life can go forward until he does what he said he would. Someone cuts in front of you in line, and you want to send her directly to the gas chamber.

You start to remember all the sadness in your life. Every hurt, every slight you've ever suffered, the way your brother teased you—you feel again as if for the first time. Suffering is your new name.

How bad can those emotions get? Oh, it's pretty astonishing just how bad they can get. What was the most depressing movie you ever saw, or story you read? Your emotions can make them seem like jokes. And the real problem is, there you are in the middle of them, unable to imagine any other possibility. You can't be objective about anything as long as you're in there. Being in your emotions is like being in a washing machine set to HEAVY.

Your parents never even wanted you to be happy, that's why they never bought you the horse/piano/ski-doo. Events in your life conspired against you. Here you are, a broken shell of a human being, violated by every circumstance in your life. Luck and good fortune have gone to others, while you spent your life struggling over one obstacle after another. Your life seems to be getting harder by the week. You're trying to cross the river by jumping from one ice floe to another, and they're getting further apart. Barricades and hurdles trip over each other to get in your way, while your so-called friends let you down when you need them, take fun trips without you, stop calling you, and take up lame hobbies you wouldn't be caught dead doing.

And what really hurts, is that you've always done the best you could. You've always tried to play fair, take care of others, keep your priorities straight, and do the right thing. You've always cared about *them*, why aren't they caring about *you*? Why aren't they here to help you, when you feel as though you can't even figure out what the *&%$ is going on?

Why does everything that happens make you hurt? How can you make anything of a day when you're feeling so much pain? Your pain, other people's pain, why is there so much of it everywhere? It seems that everywhere you look in your life, the painful parts are the only things you see. Beauty? *Ha ha.* Nothing calls to you, nothing good or fun seems likely, or even possible. Everything and everyone seem to be pushing you away, into your personal private Pit of Pain.

Things you normally enjoy don't sound interesting, going anywhere is too much trouble, doing anything is too much work. Your life spirals inward, growing smaller and smaller as you pull in all your energy, trying to protect yourself from all that pain. You pull away from anything that isn't centered on you. The world obviously doesn't need you, why should you pretend to need it?

Every argument you make, every thread of logic you try to follow leads back to itself in a circle, taking you further down into The Pit, reinforcing your desire to withdraw, to separate yourself, to hide, to rest, to be alone. Finally the tears start to come, and you cry, and cry, and cry, until you're tired of crying, until nothing is left in you with the energy to cry.

People you've loved forever suddenly develop faults you never imagined. Now it seems as though every stupid thing they do affects you. You remember slights and hurts that happened years ago that you had completely forgotten about. Every little difference that comes up seems like just one more piece of the legacy of pain between you.

Some days you mirror the pain you feel from outside, inflicting it on yourself. You tell yourself you're not good enough, you never worked hard enough, you have no talent, no abilities, no connection with anything or anyone. You walk into work and find yourself on a strange, perverse planet where people are only there to poke fun at you. Feeling good is something you've forgotten how to do; it simply doesn't have a place in your life. Your whole being is consumed with this weight of NOTHING, of not doing, of not being. Imagine a giant boneless chicken. That's how much energy you have. A lump of lead. A load of wet laundry, stuck to the inside of the wash tub. That's what you are—unmade, unmotivated, unmovable.

And then the next day, you wake up and things seem perfectly normal. You look back and see that it's been three or four days since you felt alive, and you wonder what the heck was that? What was that all about? Why did you have to go through that? Why does it keep happening?

> *The Second Law Of Menopause:* **Don't make decisions while you are in your emotions.**

If there's a decision to be made when you're not feeling calm and objective, ask for time to think about it. If that doesn't work, demand time to think about it. Say something like, "I have to think about that." "I can't give you an answer on that right now." "I'll call you tomorrow." "I have to check with my (calendar, friend, husband, kids, parents, lawyer, spiritual advisor, accountant, analyst, bookie)." Do not be pushed, harried, threatened, cajoled, enticed, or seduced.

If this is an important decision, you have every right to take time to think about it, to make a list of pros and cons, and to get advice if you want it. Make yourself the important one here, just long enough to feel cool with your choice. Remember, you are entitled to this time.

> ***The Third Law Of Menopause:*** **Let go of the past.**

Your past does have an important place, but not in your future. For better or for worse, your vacillating hormone levels are going to keep throwing every emotion you've ever felt (including some you don't remember) in your face. So that's what menopause becomes—an opportunity to release them, to let them go.

Some things you can fix, all these years later. Some things you can talk to others about, or find information on in books or on the web. Terrible things that happened to you, things you regret having done to others. Some hurts you can heal by expressing them—writing, drawing, talking, or yelling in your car as you're driving alone down the freeway.

But if you fight with those memories, resist them, argue with them, they'll come back time and again to torment you. Embrace them, accept them, forgive yourself and others as much as you possibly can, and it's amazing how many painful scars evaporate and disappear, never to return.

I believe we're here to learn, and the fact is, you don't really learn by doing things right. You learn by making mistakes, and by being affected by the mistakes of others. Learn what you can from it, then let it go. Laughing and crying about it help a lot.

Life is a stream, carrying you. There are rocks in the stream, and from time to time you hit one. If you hold onto the rock, you stop moving forward, and the stream pounds on you, wearing you down. Let go of the rock and let the stream carry you on. Wave goodbye to the past. Don't worry—you'll never lose the good stuff.

PRIORITY THREE: YOUR MIND

What happened to the woman who never forgot anything important? Whose job it was to keep everyone else on track? One minute ago you knew exactly what you wanted to say at this pause in the conversation, why can't you remember it now, when everyone is looking at you expectantly? Your jokes only have half of the punch line, and people's expressions look as though they are getting worried about you. You buy the big package of sticky notes and start writing down your onesie-twosie shopping items, only to forget to read your list when you get inside the store.

Even when you feel physically well and your emotions are balanced, you need to understand that your memory can seriously let you down. You've forgotten something important, and unfortunately the universe neglected to remind you. Something came up and pulled you in another direction and you forgot completely about it, so now you're unhappy with yourself. As often as not, people were counting on you for that, and you let them down too. Oops. Now they're angry with you too, and you feel terrible, horrible about it. It's not as if you meant to forget it, so how is that fair?

I'm tempted to believe that spending the second half of our lives forgetting things must have some kind of great cosmic significance. It does happen to everyone over the age of fifty (sometimes earlier), and there is no way to escape it, so it makes sense that it would have some actual purpose. Maybe our brains just run out of room to keep stuff.

Maybe all that dark matter in the universe, that mysterious invisible stuff that fills up the spaces between the stars, is really just a mass of thoughts, the mental lint of all those things we had to remember in our youth—silly rhymes, secret names, birthdays, directions, homework assignments, chores—you name it.

Maybe if we kept accumulating that stuff our whole lives we would get to a point where we couldn't think at all. Maybe erasing those things in our minds helps make room in the universe for the people who come along after us.

No, I don't have any clever solution for forgetting, but a wise man once told me, "When your memory starts to go—forget it."

Was today a day of mistakes? Write them down, and maybe you'll never have to make them again. Did that thing you felt that you absolutely had to try, fall through today? Write about it. Clarify why you chose to do it in the first place. Decide to try again, or choose a new plan. Are you having insights now about how you weren't reaching for exactly what you wanted? Write them down, and congratulate yourself for your growing wisdom.

The things you learned today will strengthen you tomorrow, and the things you understand tomorrow you'll pass on to someone else who can benefit from them. You are part of the endless chain of growth that is the whole of Humanity, crawling its way up the mountain. Even when you think you've failed, you're still doing your part.

> *The Fourth Law Of Menopause:* **Learn to laugh at yourself.**

You will be endlessly entertained. All of the dorky, goofy, nerdy, confused and inexplicable things that you find yourself doing, humanity has been doing since the first humans began to think they were pretty smart. It will be really great for everyone when someday we actually do get smart enough to not mess up the simplest things, but don't hold your breath. Besides, laughing is one of the most completely beneficial activities known.

If you forget something, and it really is important in a cosmic sense, the universe will remember it for you. Either a reminder will come, just in time, or others will pick it up and take care of it. You can thank them—they did you two favors: They did something you thought was your responsibility, and they let you know that you're not alone. You're not the only one carrying the burden of Life. We're all in here together.

PRIORITY FOUR: YOUR SPIRIT

You begin to mentally populate The Place Of Eternal Suffering with everyone who gets in your way. Your sense of perfect justice is that everyone has to become just like you, no one should ever do anything you wouldn't, and you are absolutely certain that you're right about that.

You take all the people you know and mentally give them the complete laundry list of personal improvements they need to make to meet your standards, and if they choose not to, well, let's see, what should they have to do? I know—they have to apologize to you. That's the only way they get to stay on Earth.

But maybe today starts out like a good day, everything happens the way it's supposed to, everyone is fine, and you have no complaints. Except...something in your life seems empty, vacant, missing. As if there were an unopened door somewhere, some chance you missed, how many years ago? What if you had done _____ instead? Or gone to _____ when you had the chance? Why did you never pick up that book/paintbrush/job/plane ticket/blonde when it/he/she came into your life? Are you really doing what you were meant to be doing? Or was there something else that might make you feel more accomplished, more satisfied, more complete right now?

> *The Fifth Law Of Menopause:* **Be grateful for all that you are, and all that you have.**

Although it may not feel like it sometimes, it's a privilege to be alive on this planet. Everything that happens in your life is an opportunity for you—to experience, to learn, to grow, to understand, to give and receive love. I know it doesn't seem that way when your body betrays you, you don't feel any support anywhere, and you can't remember the last time you were really happy. But it's true. There is a bigger, deeper part of you than your body, mind, and emotions.

A great thing about menopause is that you've lived here long enough to get to where you really see just how complicated, paradoxical and unexpected this parade of activity we know as Life *is*. You owe yourself a huge debt of gratitude for sticking around this long, to find out about all the things you never had a chance to encounter and explore in your youth.

Every day you live, you become wiser. Now is the time in your life when that wisdom grows great enough for you to put it to work. That continuously growing wisdom inside you is the payback for all the physical, mental, and emotional work you've done. And that is no small thing.

Extra credit realization: Feeling true gratitude for your life won't doom you to more of the same; it will instead bring ever more new and wonderful experiences to you.

Sleep is important because:

When you get enough SLEEP you

can RELAX and when you're

relaxed you find it easy to LAUGH

and when you're laughing you can

APPRECIATE

everything you have and everything you are.

The feelings

Not every unpleasant emotion you'll experience has a deeper meaning, or should trigger you into self-analysis. Sometimes as your hormone levels wax and wane, emotional states bubble up for no apparent reason and disappear as quickly as they came. Like an attack of gas, it can be embarrassing if it happens when you're with company, but you can learn to recognize the symptoms. After all, you had periods for how many years? Apologize if it's appropriate, forgive yourself and carry on. If something comes up more than once, or you feel you need to deal with it, make an appointment with yourself for later, and give yourself permission to take whatever time you need to work through it.

What is "working through" a feeling? It's being able to acknowledge it, to understand all sides of it, decide what to do about it, and take steps to deal with it to reach a satisfactory conclusion. Depending on the feeling, that might mean anything from laughing it off or feeling sorry for yourself for a while, to making a life-changing decision like moving to another country. Or planet.

So how do you start that process?

1.   Get as detailed as you can about what and how you're feeling. The goal is to be sure what you *are* feeling.

2. Ask yourself questions—Who? What? Since when? Be your own detective.

3. Focus on you—on *your* feelings, on *your* reactions, why this is important to *you*, and how it impacts *your* life.

4. Express your anger, your frustration, your anxiety—whatever you're feeling. If you feel like crying, go ahead and cry.

5. Accept that you have these feelings, and if any of them bother you, forgive yourself for having them.

6. Embrace yourself in your heart, choose to let go of this issue, and move on.

Going through these steps might take place a bit at a time. Working through emotions is like finding your way through a maze. There may be a number of ways to get through it and out the other side, but there are also places where you can get stuck. You can stay there as long as you need, but you don't need to stay there any longer than you want to. If you have something that simply will not let you resolve it right now, just put it in the UNRESOLVED box on the shelf in the back of your mind. It can wait.

I feel...

Sleepy tired

The most likely thing here is that you need more sleep. But other physical things can contribute to this, such as anemia or thyroid issues, so if you think you're getting enough Z's but you're often sleepy, tell your doctor. This is a good item to keep records on.

Your body and your brain do the work to keep themselves in order during your sleep, so it's vital that you get as much as you need. If that means you have to sleep half of a weekend day, you're much better off doing that than any other elective activity. It's an easy thing to deny yourself, because you expect yourself to get enough at night. Unfortunately, menopause makes that impossible for most women.

Because menopause doesn't play by the rules of polite society, you must give yourself permission to bend the rules, even break them. Remember, getting enough sleep is The Law. Your body is undergoing a great deal of change, and it needs extra time and care from you while that's happening. You won't have to do this forever. This may be why people used to think of menopause as an illness, because part of the treatment is the same—abundant rest.

At a certain age, naps become awfully attractive, especially after a big lunch. Take one if you can, it's a great way to rejuvenate. Or learn to meditate to refresh yourself during the day.

Are you losing sleep because something is keeping you awake? What keeps you awake at night? When you're lying there in the middle of the night, what is it that goes through your mind? Do you lie awake not really thinking about anything, just wishing you could go back to sleep? Is it nothing but your general, favorite worries and anxieties?

If you find that there's a particular thing that your mind keeps coming back to, it's going to be much harder to get back to sleep with it sitting at the table, banging its cup and plate, demanding your attention. Sometimes you'll have a worry or an issue come up during the day that you're able to sidestep and suppress with activity or distraction. But now it's three in the morning, you have no more excuses, and your need for sleep doesn't matter! This *thing* has a stranglehold on your attention and keeps you hostage until you deal with it.

It might be something on your conscience, or perhaps some type of new idea that's trying to break through, to get you to look at something in a different way. Stop resisting and face up to it. Cry, whine, or scream, but accept that it's there, and deal with it now. If you need help dealing with it, admit that you need help.

Want to know why this is coming up now? Because it's important for you to take care of this so you can get on with your life. You know the saying, "Timing is everything"? This issue is an obstacle to your present growth, and it's unquestionably beneficial for you to deal with it now. Decide how you'll deal with it. Now. Then give yourself a big hug for being your own best friend, and make a note that you're now officially sleep deprived, and you'll need to make it up as soon as you can.

Things to do:

1.   If getting enough sleep becomes a regular problem for you, this is something you need to take care of. Your sleep is too important to your health to let it be compromised.

2.   If you're not sure if you're getting enough sleep, keep track of how many hours you get a night.

3.   Record what kept you awake when you wanted to go back to sleep. See the worksheet on 'Midnight Thoughts'.

4.   When you want to take a nap and something gets in the way, write down what got in the way.

Because menopause doesn't play by the rules of polite society, you must give yourself permission to bend the rules, even break them. Remember, getting enough sleep is The Law.

Achy tired

You start noticing how you don't feel generally as good as you used to. You're getting little aches and pains in your back or hips or shoulders, or you feel as if your muscles are sore from exercise, only you haven't *been* exercising. You get winded going up stairs, and you really don't feel like doing any of the physical activities you used to do. You spend more time sitting or lying down than you ever did, and yet feel tired most of the time.

Years ago, you could run around all day and after a good night's sleep you could get up and do it all over again. Now you may have a desk job, or just spend most of your time driving others around, or talking on the phone, or working on tasks or activities that don't involve physical activity.

There can be any number of good reasons (and excuses) why you don't exercise regularly; I have many of them. What you need to realize is that you're paying a price for indulging in inactivity. Being physically active benefits your body in so many ways, it's like a medicine. It reduces stress— which will age you even faster—and it helps balance your hormones and reduces the physical effects of menopause. It stimulates and relaxes your mind, and when you can do it in a natural environment, helps you keep your connection to other living things.

Staying physically fit and active is the most direct way you can lessen the effects menopause has on your body and your emotions.

And just in case you're thinking it doesn't really make any difference if you're fit or not, it really, really *does* make a difference. If you're not getting enough exercise, your body will get progressively more achy as your muscles get more and more out of shape. As they lose condition, they won't hold your joints together properly, so there are more stresses on the cartilage, ligaments and tendons than your joints were really designed to handle. The harder it is for your joints to work properly, the sooner they'll show wear and tear.

Your body needs you to take care of it, now more than ever before. Only you can keep yourself in good physical condition. It will take effort on your part, and it will take time away from doing other things. There are tradeoffs here worth considering. Take a walk while you think them over.

Things to do:

1.   Keep records of any times you feel too much achiness, discomfort, or other unpleasant symptoms in your muscles or bones. How often does it happen? How bad does it get? How long does it last? Talk to your doctor about anything that bothers you, and also talk about exercise.

2.   Low impact exercise such as yoga, tai chi, dance, cycling, light gardening and shopping are great.

3.   If you're interested in something more strenuous, talk to your doctor and figure out a way to get yourself into shape for it. Just because you're not young anymore doesn't mean you're all the way over the hill. Don't assume that you can't take up a new physical activity that you've always wanted to try.

4.   But—there always seems to be a "but"—be thoughtful with high–impact exercise. Your body is older, and you don't have the strength and coordination you had ten or twenty years ago. Old injuries accumulate scar tissue, making new injuries easier to acquire. Use your mind to protect your body, to take care of it by making sensible choices.

5.   You don't have to choose an exercise program just because it works for someone else. Try to find activities that make *you* happy.

Your body needs
you to take good
care of it now, more
than ever before.

Out of sorts

You can't put your finger on it. It's not obviously physical, or obviously emotional. You think you got enough sleep, but the day just doesn't seem to be coming together quite right. It's sort of a light funk.

Sometimes an issue will come to you during the day, something inside that wants you to listen. Pay attention to yourself and how you feel. Treat yourself as you would treat your most cherished associate or client, your dearest friend, your beloved. Focus on yourself. Thank yourself for everything you do for yourself, your family, your work, all the people around you. Relax.

If you can find something that will make you laugh or cry, it may jog loose an emotion that's distracting you from just under the surface of your thoughts. Be ready to write down anything that comes to you, but don't feel as though you missed it, if nothing comes. Ideas come in their own time.

If the day ends with you still feeling the same, consider the possibility that you might be coming down with a minor illness. Be ready to go to bed early, and try to get a good night's sleep.

Things to do:

1. It's okay if you're less than 100% today. Give yourself an extra five or ten minutes in the morning to organize yourself. Write down the things that *must* get done.

2.   Just because it's a small, vague problem, don't ignore it. It's okay to listen to your body when it's just whispering. Wouldn't you feel good about giving a few minutes to a dear friend who was having a bad day? It's good practice to do the same for yourself.

3.   Pick a time later when you can give yourself half an hour either to rest by yourself, or to do something entertaining and slightly unusual.

4.   A few minutes of relaxed physical activity can restore normal flow of energy and make you feel better —an easy walk, a bit of tai chi, or a few stretches by yourself in the sunshine.

5.   Pamper yourself a tiny bit, do something nice for yourself that doesn't cost anything. Go to a library, sit on a park bench, watch toddlers playing, go window-shopping. Seek out bright colors and enjoy them. Listen to some of your favorite music.

Left behind

Feeling left behind by friends, or left behind by life—it makes no difference—it's painful either way. Your friends went off on an adventure without you. Maybe you knew about it but couldn't get free, or maybe you were surprised. It was something you would have wanted to do, but no one thought to ask you. Or people you love moved away, passed on, or have taken a new step in life and you cannot or do not want to go with them. You feel as though you're stuck here, by choice or by chance, and part of you went with them. Or it might be just a vague feeling that Life is going on somewhere else; things are happening, other people are busy and happy, and you're not part of it.

How serious is this feeling for you now? This is a time to ask more questions. Which bothers you more, that you're not out with your friends, or that you're not going to that particular place or activity? If it's just the activity that you're missing, that's a problem you can solve another time.

This kind of feeling left behind is really something that can happen at any time in your life, when you have an expectation that your friends will include you, and for some reason, that doesn't happen. The only reason I include this issue here is that this is the kind of normal life disappointment which during menopause can trigger several days of recriminations and pain. What you really want to do is look at what other frustrations it brings up, especially old memories.

Are you feeling a "What am I doing (or not doing) with my life" issue, as if you've somehow gotten off your path? Are you feeling as though you're running out of time to do the things you want? If either of these issues feels as if it applies to you, see the 'Midwife Your Life' worksheet.

Things to do:

1. Make sure you're not just tired. If part of you didn't show up today, you may simply need some rest.

2. What activities would you rather be doing now, in place of what's currently on your plate? Make a list and keep it up to date.

3. Pick something from that list and choose a time to do it, with or without friends.

4. Talk to one or more of your friends and make an appointment to spend some time with them.

5. Call or email someone you haven't talked to in a long time and find out how they are.

Angry

This is an unpleasant emotion to be caught in, and one you want to deal with as soon as possible. Anger cries out to be expressed. It's a fierce energy that serves a real purpose in survival situations, and can give you the courage to stand up to abuse, manipulation, or disrespect from others.

Anger is unmistakable, but sometimes we become so focused on the object of our anger that we forget that what we need to deal with is the feeling right here, inside us. Try to separate the feeling you're having from the event or person who caused it. You may not be able to do anything about the cause, but you do have power over your feelings. There are plenty of good books on anger and how to deal with it in a healthy manner. Don't hesitate to get one or more if you'd rather rule it than let it rule you.

If you can't go write about it now, and you don't want to speak out, make a plan right then to write about it later, and be sure to do it. Most of the feelings will come back up to be expressed; in fact, you might even get more. Most likely, the event that made you angry has happened before; you may have a long, long history of this kind of event. If that's the case, you can't begin soon enough to express the anger and release it.

Anger that you've held onto for a long time, anger that's built up over many occurrences, may take many times to come out completely. If you thought you had cleared something out and it comes up again, just work with it as you did the first time. Write it all out, every word of every feeling and let it go. It will stop eventually. It'll wind down to less and less emotion and eventually you'll just announce, "Oh that's enough. I'm done with that," and you will be done. And you will have had a lot of experience handling your anger in productive healthy ways. Imagine being able to deal with serious disagreement and conflict without losing your cool. You could face situations that would have frozen you before. When you have a calm mind and your wit, reason and compassion at your command, it's a lot easier to deal with whatever comes along.

Things to do:

1.   On a scale of 1 to 10, how angry are you?

2.   How many times have you been angry about this before?

3.   Does this bring up other things that have made you angry?

4.   Use your journal to write how angry you are. Write down everything you're angry about; stop at nothing. Get it all off your chest. Dispose of the pages afterward if you feel you've revealed too much. Your goal is to spit it out on paper, to write and write until it all comes out. You don't ever have to show it to anyone else. This is between you and yourself.

5.   Physical activity can help you release anger. Take it out on weeds or dust bunnies, walk or run it off. Hit golf balls or tennis balls, go to a shooting range, or beat your rugs.

Frustrated

Your progress is blocked by persons or circumstances. People don't do what you thought they would, or what they said they would. You take all the right steps, but you don't get the results you want. Maybe it's all happened before. Or you know what needs to happen, but you can't do it, and other people either cannot or will not. You have a clear picture in your head or your heart of the goal, but that is as close as you can get to it. Your hopes and expectations are unfulfilled, unsatisfied.

The more you've imagined achieving your goals, the more frustrated you are, because you have all this emotional investment in that desired outcome. It feels as though the universe reached out a big hand and pushed it square in your chest, blocking any possibility of moving forward.

Frustration must be one of the most common negative emotions. It can be so common in your life that you might feel as if your major task in life is just to accomplish the simplest things. Anyone who works to achieve progress is either frustrated constantly, or very philosophical.

Be assured that you will be able to move forward, as soon as you're able to work through your emotional reaction, including your feelings of anger and helplessness. Life will go on in one direction or another, and you'll think of something better or different to do. This is the process of living and working. Surmounting obstacles, one after another, is how all things great and small are accomplished. It's in learning how to go over, under, around and through these obstacles that we acquire our greatest skills. Don't let your emotions convince you that you've failed.

Watch out for recurring frustration that makes you feel helpless, when you feel overwhelmed by your own reactions. You get completely sucked into the idea of failure, and internalize it. Instead of making this feeling part of your regular mindset, if you can realize that this is not the end and that there *are* productive results in your future, you'll be able to keep today in perspective.

Things to do:

1.   What is it that's frustrating you? (Maybe there is a looooooong list of things...or people.)

2.   Is there a history behind this frustration?

3.   Write down all you can about the circumstances. Writing can help you include the bigger picture and see additional alternatives. It can also help you to see clearly when it's time for you to shift your energy to other tasks or pursuits.

4.   Follow up this situation by writing down how you feel about it when you feel completely calm. Note anything your intuition might be telling you.

5.   Sometimes situations take more time than you'd ever expect to become resolved. Shift your focus to another part of your life and put your energy there instead.

Helpless

Helplessness is when your personal wheels fall off. It's an emotional state of full stop, the complete inability to move forward until something changes. The brakes are stuck on or the car's in a ditch. Your mind is nailed to the floor and cannot get up. You may have gotten here by way of another emotion—frustration, anger, sadness, or feeling disconnected. Perhaps a decision is facing you, a choice between two equally undesirable things. You may be facing a problem you really don't know anything about. Or, the feeling may have come on you out of the blue and you don't know what's happening, or why.

Mentally you're staggered; you may have a million things going through your mind, or you don't know what to think. You may feel emotionally overwhelmed, or not emotional at all. Your physical state may be anything, but it's unimportant compared to your other states. Spirituality is the last thing you're going to be able to think about.

Sometimes helplessness is Nature's way of telling you that the ball really is in someone else's court. Other times you have to let go of some of your goals, and accept a compromise as the best solution for all concerned.

Just because you can't do something by yourself, that doesn't mean you can't help other people do it. Being able to work cooperatively on a task is a hugely beneficial skill.

Things to do:

1.   Note any emotions that you have. Getting a handle on how you feel can help your mind stop spinning.

2.   Do something physical; preferably something that doesn't require thought. For the moment, try not to think, but connect with your body while you're moving. Take deep relaxed breaths and focus on your movements.

3.   Once your mind feels calm and quiet, start it thinking actively again by writing your priorities. What are the most important things to you right now? Once you're clear on that, write what you'd like to have happen.

4.   Now that you have that background set down, you can objectively analyze whatever problem or difficult choice you're facing. If a new or strange idea occurs to you, don't automatically discard it.

5.   Take as much time as you can, and get as much help as you want. Other people may have ideas you won't think of. Sort their input against your priorities; make your own decision, if it's your decision to make.

6.   If you're starting to feel that you'll never accomplish anything, remind yourself of all the things that you already *have* accomplished.

Stuck waiting

In stuck waiting, something very important to you and your future is on hold due to circumstances beyond your control, and there is nothing you can do to hurry it. It might take so long to happen that you really can't be sure that it ever will. This is something that carries a lot of emotional weight with you; you might feel as if your whole future depends on it.

There are two things you have to do to move forward in your life. You have to let go of any ideas that are holding you back, and you have to move in the direction of your choice.

Being stuck waiting is very similar to the state of helplessness. I didn't understand this until a few years after menopause, although the clues were there all the time. I may have seen them, but didn't know what to do with them because I hadn't really learned how to start things on my own. So, I spent a lot of time feeling tied up emotionally—and waiting. Waiting for something outside of me to happen.

The secret to escaping stuck waiting is actually really simple: Do something else. Pick any other activity you'd like to do, to learn, or to use as a means to satisfy some other need—something as simple as taking up a hobby or sport to meet people—and do it. It's like a bonus—an activity that you otherwise would not have been able to make time for in your life. Ta-*da*! You're not stuck waiting any more! You're moving forward with your life!

<u>Things to do:</u>

1.   Acknowledge that the event or person you're waiting on really is important to you, or you wouldn't be putting yourself through this.

2.   Now note all the other emotions that having to wait is bringing up in you—frustration, resentment, anger. Work through them as much as you can. Support yourself as you do this. Your goal is to get to the other side of those feelings, not to push them down in your gut and grind them into your soul.

3.   Get out your wish list of things that you'd like to do if you had the time. Pick one, and start shifting some energy over to that. Let yourself get excited about it, and take the first steps to get into it. You are a valuable person, you know; the world can benefit in some way from every activity you put your heart into. Make the most of the time you have by putting yourself into activities you love, and getting the pleasure you deserve out of them.

Resentful

Someone dismissed you or your ideas; they were inconsiderate, rude or insulting, or interfered with something important to you. Someone or something:

- Pushes one of your "hot buttons";

- Gets something you expected to get;

- Puts you down or ignores you;

- Frustrates your goals or ambitions;

- Reminds you of all the bad things you feel about yourself.

The normal human reaction in these cases is resentment. In fact, it takes almost superhuman wisdom and understanding not to feel resentment. Not feeling resentment when stuff happens is something most people really have to work hard at doing, but anyone can learn how to release this feeling. Resentment can also come from looking outside you for the causes of your unhappiness.

Resentment is low-volume anger. Swallowed and stored, it builds to anger, to blow-ups and all the consequences that go with them. And every time you feel it, it's taking energy you could be using to do something productive. Think of it as a toxin that you're allowing into your body that'll stay there until you clear it out through letting go of the event and then understanding your reaction to it. Giving resentment a permanent place in your feelings is also throwing away your power. It's saying you have no control of yourself in this situation, that nothing you can do will improve it. It excuses you from having to accept and deal with reality.

The fact is that no matter what you want, you're going to have to figure out a way to make it happen yourself. Remember that this is *your* life! Be the architect of your own life. Choose to keep yourself relaxed, happy and healthy, regardless of what other people do.

Things to do:

1.   What other feelings did this situation bring on? Frustration? Loss or anxiety about your life or choices? Look closely at the resentment you're feeling. Take note of the situation that brings it on, and any negative feelings about yourself that it reinforces, such as helplessness, lack of self-confidence, or an inability to speak up for yourself.

2.   You can first choose whether to deal with the situation itself, or with how it bothers you. Whatever you do to respond, try to do it from a feeling of love and self-respect. The calmer you feel when you act, the better you're going to feel about the outcome. If that means waiting a bit before responding, that may be the best thing.

3.   What would have to happen for you to completely let go of this resentment?

4.   Crank up your creativity and imagine a part of yourself devising a personal shield for you that would keep you from ever being bothered in these circumstances again.

Just plain grumpy

Temporary grumpiness is so often due to a physical issue that it's probably the first cause you should think of. You didn't get enough sleep, or the right amount of caffeine. You may have physical pain that you're pushing aside and trying to ignore—headache, backache, or cramps. You may be physically, mentally or emotionally exhausted. Without thinking, you're taking out your pain on others as a defense mechanism, simply because you don't have the energy to interact with them. "Leave me alone" is the unspoken message you're radiating.

The second most common cause is recent unresolved hurt or anger. Your porcupine spines are up and anyone who comes close is going to get poked. It's impersonal and universal. The third possibility is that for some cosmic reason, some old pain is coming up for you to deal with. Maybe it's the hormones du jour, or some more spiritual reason, but it's been handed to you now and you have to deal with it.

This is a really good time to be your own best friend. If you can get away from people for fifteen minutes, see if you can figure out what the cause is. If you're tired or in pain, ask if you can borrow a smile or laugh from someone you're close to. A little bit of empathy from a friend can help you feel a lot better, and give you that tiny bit of energy you need to hang on until you can go take care of yourself.

But do go take care of yourself as soon as you can. Remember that *your* health and happiness have a high priority. Take a nap, take a pain remedy, go see a doctor. If it's an unresolved anger issue, remind yourself that it's really coming from something else you need to work through, and deal with that when you can. In a busy office setting, one unkind, angry flare-up can ricochet from person to person for hours, hurting one set of feelings after another, wasting energy and slowing down everything.

If you're dealing with an emotion that's so big it's keeping you from functioning, treat it as you would a physical injury, and go take care of it. Trust that there is a reason that this is coming up for you now. Now is the time for you to start working on it.

Things to do:

1. Relax. Give yourself a real hug.

2. Want to cry? Go find someplace private and cry.

3. If you're getting blindsided frequently by emotional upwellings, think about how you can make room in your daily schedule for some amount of unpredictability. The only productive thing you can do with these events is deal with them as they come up, the same as you would with a physical problem. This is a new phase in your life, and it'll need to be accommodated.

Rushed

This is another one of those pressures that will happen throughout your life. The problem with it happening during menopause is that when your body and emotions are screaming at you that you have no control over anything at all, any extra pressure can send you right around the bend. Do everything you can to relax.

Take care of the most important things first, and if something has to fall off your schedule, then it has to fall off. *Rescheduling happens*; do it as soon as you find out you need to. The same rule applies here as for forgetting. If something is really important, the universe will pick it up.

If not having enough time is getting to be a common problem for you, it's a good time to do some long range prioritizing. You may have to let some things—and maybe some people too—pass out of your life. There may be repercussions you'll have to deal with from family or friends who have been used to getting more of your time and attention. Trust your feelings, but be sure to take care of yourself.

Don't give up the time you need for yourself. During menopause, you need to give yourself a higher priority.

Things to do:

1.   Whenever time comes up as an issue, it's always a good idea to go back to your priorities.

2.   If your job offers time management training, take advantage of it. This is a life skill everyone can use.

3.   Next time you're in a bookshop or an online bookseller, look through some of the books on time management and see if one might give you some ideas.

4.   Keep a schedule calendar, and keep it up to date. Use it to plan your month, your week and your day. It'll help keep you from piling up too much stuff at any one time.

5.   You can't stay busy all day, every day, and not expect to slow down *and* get behind. Schedule your own downtime into that calendar.

Harassed

Is there someone in your life who's giving you a bad time? Is there someone who really seems to have it in for you? Maybe it's an extended family member you have a long history with, or maybe someone you don't know well, or a new coworker. Their comments seem unnecessarily blunt or negative, or you feel as though they're judging you.

The people with whom you live and work and interact are part of your environment, and they have a powerful impact on your quality of life. As an adult, you have some power to change from an unsupportive, negative environment to a positive, supportive one, but there will always be difficult people, and there will always have to be compromises in dealing with them—unless you become a hermit. Once you decide to take charge of your happiness even with unpleasant people, then it becomes a matter of understanding how you react to them, and making whatever changes you can to lessen or remove their impact on you.

During menopause, this is another type of unhappy situation that can be taken all out of proportion when you're in your emotions. Try to keep it in perspective. Whether you decide to confront them directly, or try through friends to learn more about them, try to make that decision when you're calm and feeling centered. Don't jump to conclusions, and remember—other people are their own problem. It's not your job to change or fix them.

If you can learn to tolerate other people's faults and foibles, you will definitely be more calm. You don't need to embrace them, necessarily, but just writing them off as a circumstance of nature, like a crack in the sidewalk you have to step over, can help you adapt to their presence. There may be nice people you'd enjoy knowing behind those unpleasant facades, or they might be right bastards and all you can do is be grateful you don't have to interact with them any more than is absolutely necessary. In any case, the goal is to not let them get in the way of you being happy, healthy, and living your life the way you want to live it.

The long-term solution is to be strong within yourself, have confidence in yourself and your life, and treat negative people as you would anything else that's bad for you. If you take the attitude that even bad things are there in your life for you to learn from, then you always win.

Things to do:

1. Love yourself unconditionally.

2. How does this person make you feel bad? Describe to yourself what happens, and the feelings you go through.

3. If you find yourself repeatedly asking "Why?" or trying to analyze this person's behavior, shift your focus back to yourself, and to your own feelings. What is this situation bringing up in you?

Unappreciated

I have no doubt that things you do go unappreciated, and that you as a person are underappreciated. Very few of us are truly sufficiently appreciated by our family, companions and peers. No one knows you as well as yourself and knows how much effort you put into your work, or the special care you take for the people and things that you love. You probably have talents and abilities you've hidden from even your closest friends for years, maybe just for lack of time to pursue them. It happens far too commonly that we hide our deepest interests and feelings, when those that are the deepest are the most likely to be felt by others. And it's sad that we fail to share our gifts with others, for fear that they won't appreciate or value them as we do.

It may only happen as we get older and acquire more social skills and have less fear of rejection that we learn how to find a receptive audience for our secret, cherished gifts. Do you appreciate your own talents and inborn abilities? Do you take time to nourish them, to find ways to use them in your life? To develop them and grow your own confidence in them? Do you realize how important it is that you have those gifts? Would you enjoy making it one of your life tasks to find ways either to use them for your own benefit or share them with the world?

What is appreciation, but love expressed? When you say you want to be appreciated, do you mean you want to feel love? A thank-you, a smile, taking someone's hand, a hug, a moment taken to share a feeling of mutual happiness—how many different ways do you show your appreciation? These are the things that feed our souls and make our lives worth living.

Like water flowing through a pipe, love has to flow to be felt. It's only felt when it's given or received. The fortunate thing about love is that you feel it just as much when you're giving it as when you're getting it. You can double or triple the love you feel in a day by expressing the appreciation you feel for others.

Take the smallest excuse to say thank you, to smile and acknowledge people, and to let them feel your appreciation. You don't have to make a big deal of it—if you feel it, they will. Say good morning with a heartfelt smile, and silently wish the people around you well. Do it till you feel the love in your heart, and let it flow out to them. You don't have to stop there; you can give thanks every day for everyone and everything you love in your life. Let your love flow out to all those things, and you'll feel love rushing into you like a flood. People will get accustomed to your good will, and you'll get those smiles you want from them, those thank-yous that you need, because you give so freely of them.

If you've been expecting others to recognize or acknowledge something you did or said, stop waiting for them —give yourself the recognition you desire and deserve. Tell yourself what an interesting, accomplished, supportive and generous person you are. Think of something about yourself that you especially like and appreciate. Give thanks for that gift, and for your effort to use it and share it.

You have one supreme obligation with regard to appreciation: You must appreciate everything you are—all your gifts, all your flaws, all your strengths and weaknesses alike. You are too precious, too important, not to appreciate yourself as no other human can. Love everything you are, and everything you do. Everything in your life has meaning and significance, and you must remember that. That must be your guiding principle for everything you think and feel about yourself. You're the perfect example of yourself, you're the only one of you in this world, and you're here for many reasons. Be glad for everything you can do, and be the first to acknowledge in your heart everything you accomplish, every lesson you learn, every bit of understanding that you acquire. Know that you are exactly what you are meant to be, doing exactly what you are meant to do.

Things to do:

1. Tell yourself right now how much you appreciate yourself.

2. Acknowledge all the love and effort you put into your life. Keep a list because you're not going to be able to remember it all.

3. When others seem to go above and beyond the norm, or do anything to make your life simpler or easier, tell them how much you appreciate that, or give them a really heartfelt thank-you. That just might make their day.

4. Celebrate every job well done, whether it's yours or someone else's. Think of it as letting the universe know what you like.

5. Make sure the people in your life who provide anything for you know that you appreciate them. It won't take much effort on your part, and think how much it means to you when you get that kind of feedback.

Appreciate everything you are —all your gifts, all your flaws, all your strengths and weaknesses alike.

Abandoned

The abandoned feeling is like Left Behind, only on a more global scale. You're not just trying to figure out how to catch up, you're trying to figure out where you are, and where you belong. It's like slipping and falling and not being able to tell where you landed.

Feeling abandoned is basically a rite of passage during menopause. It's the one ride at the fair that *everyone* has to take. That doesn't make it any less important, and it may be accompanied by a major life-altering event. There are many things that can make any woman, including you, feel abandoned at this time in her life. Your family may be fragmenting. Your kids may be moving away, going away to school, going out on their own, finding their own partners and not wanting you for much of anything.

At the extreme end of the scale, your marriage or sexual relationship may be ending. You may have been laid off from your job, or lost a family member, best friend or respected coworker. The main threads of your life for the last twenty or thirty years may be loosening and pulling away, leaving you with big empty places to fill. No one can go through any of those without feeling abandoned.

Or maybe your life is not changing right now, but the way you feel about it is. Let's go back to the whole reason for menopause—your body is losing its ability to produce babies. Nature thinks you're too old to be a good birth mother. You are losing your biogenic potential. So, barring a miracle, you've had your chance to pass on your genes to the population, and that portion of your life is over. In that sense, life is moving on without you; it's abandoning you as a candidate for motherhood.

As you get further into menopause and the changes in you start to accumulate, you may begin to feel that you've turned into a different person than you were before. As you cast off the restrictions and assumptions of your past that don't apply any more, you can find yourself picking up threads of dreams from your childhood, or coming up with dreams that you never imagined before.

No matter what you've been doing for the last few decades, you've probably acquired a lot more skills than even your friends know you have. What if you could do work that would give you a chance not only to do things you really believe in, but also to make use of your special talents and skills? Now that you're finally a grown-up, that's not necessarily impossible, is it?

You may have half of your adult life expectancy still ahead of you. Think about what more you'd need to get started doing something that you never had the time or the resources to work on before. You can turn your own growth and development into a major project.

Things to do:

1. Yearn to learn. Pick *anything* and learn something new about it.

2. Do some abandoning yourself: give yourself the right to abandon things that don't work for you any more in favor of those that do.

3. Turn your imagination loose on your desires.

4.   Practice visualizing yourself in your future. Be open to any nice surprises that come up.

5.   Practice something like this: "These are the things I choose to believe about myself...."

6.   Believe that anything is possible where your dreams are concerned.

7.   If you're thinking, "I need to figure out what I should do," change that to, "I need to figure out what I really want to do."

Cast off the restrictions and assumptions of your past that don't apply to you any more.

Disconnected

The places and activities you spend time in, the people you relate to and can be yourself with—those are your connections to the lives and activities around you. Your higher connections, at a spiritual level, are the things that give your life meaning beyond physical relationships and existence. These are the grit and grist of our daily lives—those things we act on, and those that act on us. That's what I mean by connections.

When you feel disconnected, it's just as if someone unplugged you from the switchboard. You can't remember why any of those things are important. Part of it is feeling as though you have no energy to interact with any of them, but there is also a sense that even if you had energy, you have no reason or purpose to care about any part of your life right now. If it's a place, you have no reason to go, if it's a thing, it gives you no pleasure nor can it do you any good, if it's an activity, you make a face and say, "Nawwwwww, I don't wanna...."

The clue is that all these things are a normal part of your life and you usually care about what's going on with them, but right now you would rather stare at a wall than have anything to do with any of them. You're disconnected from your life. It's like watching a movie on a very small screen with the sound turned off.

Part of the process of growing and evolving is that every now and then we go through what I call "shifts." They're times when things seem to stand still for a bit, and I'm never sure whether the world has to catch up with me, or I need to catch up with it. Usually these out-of-sync periods just last a day or so.

It may be a perfect storm of hormones that does a big reset of your emotional self, or maybe your self just needs to turn down the volume on your emotions so it can focus on other things. Take this time to turn inward, to pay attention to yourself.

Things to do:

1.   Are you exhausted, physically or emotionally? Do you feel as though you're in an intermission?

2.   Are you facing a crisis, or even just a major event right now? Something so big that it's taking all your mental capacity to deal with it? If so, it's perfectly normal for all your emotional energy as well to be focused on that. Take it easy.

3.   What is your body saying right now? If it's tired, take care of it. Remember, nothing works well when you're tired.

4.   Think about what an amazing being you are, all of the hundreds of small and large things you've accomplished in your life. Remember that no one else in the world has the unique combination of qualities, abilities and hard-won skills you have. You are a being of infinite potential. At this time, when other things seem so uninteresting and far away, spend some time with the miracle that is you.

5.   What would you like the essence of your life to be?

6. If there were one question you could ask right now, and know that you'd get the answer, what would you ask?

7. If there were a door in front of you right now, and a mystery behind it, would you want to open it right now? What would you like to find there?

When other things
seem uninteresting
and far away, spend
some time with the
miracle that is you.

Betrayed

You feel as though part of your most secret, private self has been spread out on a billboard for all to see. You feel exposed in the worst possible way, your personal laundry hung out to dry with no way for you to ever pull it back in and hide it again. Your personal security, the boundary you put up around you and your private life, has been violated in a way that leaves you feeling way too vulnerable for comfort. It could cause you embarrassment or complications, put your job or significant relationship at risk, or just be really irritating because you consider that part of your life to be nobody else's business.

Events like betrayal always take you by surprise, and there lies the big problem. Whatever happens now happens to some extent in front of an audience whom you wish were on another planet right now. I'm guessing this is not your idea of a good time. This feeling really hits a lot of hot buttons and will bring up every fear and anxiety you have about yourself, every self-confidence issue you've ever had.

Betrayal is one of the more subtle, complicated feelings you can get slapped with. It might take a few days to get any insights about this experience. Don't feel that you have to jump to any conclusions.

Exposures of one's private self are a particularly abrupt way the universe has of dealing with our egos as well as our secrets. While they are painful and may leave you feeling destroyed in some fashion, it's better to look at them as an assumption you made on faulty evidence, which the universe has taken the trouble to correct. It's time to adjust yourself to this new, resulting reality. While it may be difficult, possibly life changing, it's healthier, and it's actually important for you in a way that only you can find or figure out. In the long run, the circumstances of the exposure and the personalities involved are less important than how you choose to integrate this new reality into your outlook.

Things to do:

1.   The key to dealing with this situation is first to keep your perspective when it happens. If it's a relatively small thing and you can laugh it off, that gives you an immediate out and you can take the wheelbarrow of your emotional responses off to somewhere private where you can deal with them. If on the other hand there *is* something serious going on, the calmer you are right now, the more intelligently you can deal with it.

2.   Before you work with your emotions, do triage first. Remember that there is much more to you as a person and human being than this newly revealed concern. Remember that you're a whole, healthy, marvelous woman, and all these emotions you're feeling right now are a normal response to what happened.

3.   As soon as you can get away, write, say, or scream all the feelings you're having, with all the gory details. Express what the possible outcome is that you're afraid might happen, or any regrets you're feeling. Let it all come out.

Alone

It happens in the middle of a conversation, or a meeting, or you're in the car with your family. Suddenly you have a feeling that there is no one "with" you. While they're not quite pod people, all the people around you seem focused on each other. They don't ask you how you are; they don't ask you anything. They're talking about themselves, or something you have no interest in. Or maybe they're telling you what you should do, what you should think, what you should care about. You feel as though you might as well be in a glass box. You might have no feeling about it, or you might be bored, or you might wish that someone, anyone, wanted to be in the space you're in right now.

But did they drift away, or did you? When something comes up from your memories, or your mind just jumped on a recent issue as if it's the only thing in the world, you may need your own company for a bit. There may be some part of you that wants right now to be heard, to be asked how you feel, that really wants to have a best friend be there for you right now. So why is no one else doing that for you, when it's so important to you? Promise yourself some time for this later, and steer your mind back to the present moment.

One survival skill you can develop is the ability to ask for what you truly need, when you need it. People need both solitude and companionship; your feelings will tell you which you need at any point in time. You need to listen to those feelings, and you need to act on them.

Things to do:

1.   In an emergency, act as your own best friend and ask yourself questions to explore your feelings, get things off your chest, and release any emotions that you've been saving up on the back burner. What would the ideal sympathetic friend be asking you right now? What do you most want to say?

2.   It may be harder during menopause to ignore your inner activities, and you may experience conflicting demands from your self and your friends. You need time with both. If you have to say no to either one, try to make up that time as soon as you can.

3.   Most minds love to wander off. La la la la la la la la la. This is your mind on roller skates. Your mind belongs to you, not the other way around. Make it do what you want.

4.   We need friends because everyone needs someone else to connect with, sometimes. If you have a need right now to feel close to someone, call your best friend and ask her if she has time to talk. If she's not available right then, either make an appointment to spend time with her or call the next person on your list.

5.   Know your support group. They're an important factor in your health and happiness. Take care of them and let them take care of you when you need it. You deserve it.

6.   How good are you at asking for help?

Physically sick

I'm guessing you already know what it feels like to be sick; you've probably had illnesses before in your forty or more years in your body. However, you can have new or unfamiliar physical feelings during menopause that are persistent enough, strange enough, or strong enough that you're not sure if they indicate an illness or not. Parts of your body may be aching—muscles and joints, your gut, your chest, different areas of your back.

Write your physical symptoms down in your journal. If any of them are starting to bother you, ask your doctor about them. Discuss how often and how significant the symptoms are. Get help until you figure out what it is.

Things to do:

1.   Think of your body as something you absolutely cannot live without. Duh. Don't take it for granted.

2.   If you have a question about something your body is doing, make it your homework to find out about it. Books, the web, any doctor you have access to, classes, support groups, friends—especially friends in menopause—all these can help you find the answers you're looking for. Don't jump to conclusions, keep researching till you're satisfied, and bounce your thoughts off your doctor. If you don't get an answer that makes sense to you, ask where to take your research next; whom else can you talk to? Institutions, research facilities, university hospitals?

3.   If you're sick, take care of yourself, and don't hesitate to call your doctor if you think you might need to. Never be afraid to ask for help. Don't think that being the responsible caregiver means you don't have to take care of yourself. Remember that in airplanes when the oxygen masks drop down, they always tell you to put yours on first before you take care of anyone else. It's the same with your body. You're not any good to anyone if you lose it.

Sad

Sadness is an emotion asking for your time and attention. Whatever it is that's making you sad isn't just anything—it's something you care about. If you can't deal with it right now, make an appointment with yourself to spend some time to come to peace with it. Use whatever tools of expression you need to express and validate your feelings. No matter how trivial the object or occasion seems, there's a reason you have this feeling.

In a way, sadness is a sign of growth. As we learn to care for more things outside ourselves, it's part of life that we will suffer loss. Whether we lose something or someone we love, or some part of the way we're used to looking at the world, the cuts go deep enough to need healing. Your affections and attachments are literally part of you, both mentally and emotionally. Your sadness deserves to be honored.

Some issue you're holding inside needs to be addressed. Grieving the loss of something important to you is part of the process you need in order to heal. This pain is part of the human condition, and nothing about feeling sadness should make you feel there is something wrong with you. Acknowledge it as simply, respectfully, and quickly as you can, then let go of it and move on. If it comes back, work with it again, and look for connections to other previous losses that also need to be acknowledged and dealt with.

There are still a lot of people in the world who don't believe that emotions are real; for me they're completely real. I view an emotional attachment as an energy connection to someone or something, just like a cord or cable that is tied to my body. To me, that's what an attachment is. When the thing or person at the other end of the cord goes away, I feel loss and sadness until that break heals. Sometimes a loss is so big it seems to have dozens of those cords, and it can take years for all of them to come to the surface to be healed. Be patient with yourself. All you can do is what you can do.

Another kind of loss that can really hurt is an unrealized expectation. The downside of having a fertile imagination is that you can use it to create an incredibly detailed and attractive outcome that seems completely possible yet has no foundation whatsoever in reality. Every part of this imaginary creation that you invest with emotion is going to have exactly the same painful attachments as all the real things you love. When one of these lovely daydreams dies, give it at least a token funeral.

Things to do:

1. Remind yourself that you have a right to feel sad about losing something important to you. Understand that it may take you some time to adjust completely to this loss.

2. Write what it was about that thing that was important to you, what you received or learned or expected from it.

3. If it was someone close to you who passed and you're having trouble coming to terms with their passing, consider doing something to honor them or your relationship. That could be anything from a public

donation to a secret memorial, but it'll be something in the world that embodies the affection you feel.

4. Crying and laughing are equally effective at releasing sadness and helping you integrate loss. Sometimes it's hard to get started; use a trigger such as a movie, a memory, or physical activity. Let it all come out.

5. There is a belief that going through the sadness of loss increases our ability for joy. That may just seem like a rationalization for pain, but I think it's true. There is no doubt that trying to avoid ever being sad, pushing down your sad feelings, or blocking or denying them are all major joy killers that can make you miss out on many of the great events of living.

6. Don't ever think that we're not supposed to care. We're *built* to care.

7. There are many spiritual lessons in sadness. Besides helping us to learn how to handle change, it also teaches us to appreciate the things and people that we do have in our lives.

Your affections and
attachments are
literally part of you,
both mentally and
emotionally.

Sorry

Being sorry, feeling regret after realizing and acknowledging that you've done something inappropriate, stupid, or dangerous, is part of a very important process of living. It's part of learning from our actions and the actions of others. Be glad when you have this feeling, it's a very good sign that you're getting smarter. You've endured the painful consequences of an unfortunate choice, and now you know a really good reason not to make that choice again, at least under the same circumstances. This is how most of us acquire knowledge, most of the time.

If it was a really painful or embarrassing consequence, then you've also probably picked up a bit of compassion for others who have made the same choice. Congratulations— you're human. And, you're becoming a more wise and compassionate human every day. Apologize—to yourself as well—make it better if you can, and move on to your next lesson. With luck, that one will be more fun.

Doing things we regret teaches us about forgiveness. Learning to truly forgive yourself is a really practical skill, because learning how to forgive others is critical to ever having long-term healthy relationships. People hurt each other all the time, whether they want to or not. It's a natural consequence of living and growing, and it's all tied up with learning to accept yourself the way you are, and others just the way they are.

Self-forgiveness is not about saying that what happened was "okay." It means that you recognize you did something that wasn't good, wasn't right or wasn't fair, and if you had it to do over, you'd want to do it differently. It means you learned something useful from what happened. It's not only healthy for you to admit these things, it's in everyone's highest and best interests, especially yours.

Things to do:

1.   If you're feeling sorry about something you said or did, the quickest way to feel better is to apologize for it.

2.   Let the apology come from your heart.

3.   Forgive everyone who was involved, and then forgive yourself completely. Say to yourself, "I forgive myself completely for what I did."

Guilty

This one usually comes before Sorry, doesn't it? It's the secret stage, the one where you know something bad happened, but don't quite feel the regret yet. Whatever happened, you feel it was your fault. Guilt is another sign of growth, just not so far along. Sometimes it takes some objectivity to really see how everything happened and be clear on your role in it, but this is a hard one to get feedback on because you really aren't ready to talk about it to anyone. This is like the "simmer" stage, where you need to cook in your own juices until all the relevant pieces come together. If no one else is going to blow the whistle on you, and you're not ready to talk about it, this stage could last for a while.

Most of us learn the technique of pushing this one under the rug by the time we leave childhood, which is too bad. Guilt does accumulate, and it's not doing you any good while it's accumulating. It's sucking energy out of you, making knots in your gut, blocking off parts of your mind with little emotional barriers to keep you from going there. If ever there was a waste of brain cells, this is it. If you're having trouble seeing how a problem that you seem to have created can become a powerful lesson, writing it down can really help you see the whole big picture.

Carrying around long-held guilt is like having a parasite on your energy source. You can't afford that any more, remember? You need every bit of energy you have just to keep yourself healthy and deal with your other menopause symptoms and the rest of your activities. Do yourself and everyone in your life a favor, and work through this. The goal is to let it go. That doesn't necessarily mean that it was fine for you to do it, but it does mean it's time for you to face it, make amends at whatever level you can, and learn from it.

This is so important, I'm going to say it for a second time: Making mistakes is how we learn what not to do. It's how we become fully realized human beings. There is no way to avoid it, so the sooner you learn how to accept and forgive your own errors, the less time it'll take you to become the person you're capable of being. See *Sorry*.

Things to do:

1. Confess it to yourself, if you can't confess it to anyone else. Writing about guilt is very useful because it seems to really help you see the entire event in perspective. If you have to, shred the paper afterwards. At this point, you might be the only one who cares any more about this issue.

2. In the act of sorting it all out, you may find things that you really don't think you had any control over, and shouldn't have any guilt feelings about. Surprise! Something else is going on here, isn't it? What was it that made you feel in the first place that this part was your fault?

3. If you do start feeling responsibility and regret, don't be afraid to take it to the next step. No sane adult ever gets off this planet without spending some time in the "Sorry" room.

None of the above

Isn't it wonderful to have a day, or an hour, or a few minutes where nothing is bothering you? These are the moments we go through all that other stuff for. Take a deep breath, love yourself, and give thanks for the magnificent, amazing, delightful person you are, and for how much you have grown.

Things to do:

1.   Mentally wrap your arms around everything in your life and hold it all next to your heart, just for a moment.

2.   Appreciate all the people you love and benefit from.

3.   Remember that it was all those lessons you've lived through that make you the wonderful, loving, understanding person you are.

4.   Look for a moment of magic in your day.

5.   Follow an intriguing impulse.

6.   Write down anything funny or meaningful you think of.

7.   Do something to charge your personal batteries.

8.   Give yourself a hug and tell your body how much you love having it.

9.   Imagine the face of someone you love giving you a big smile.

Doing things you love will charge up your personal batteries.

It feels as if...

I can't remember where I left my brain

The bad news is, your brain is aging, and you're going to have to work harder than you used to if you want to stay on top of all the things you need to remember. The good news is that there are different techniques you can use to exercise and train your memory and keep it performing well, and ways to provide yourself with a backup system to keep you on track.

There are hundreds of books, videos and workshops on how to train your memory...if you can remember to get one of them. You can start developing your own backup system of notes, emails, and voicemails. You will forget things, and that's all there is to it. Now, what was I going to say?

Besides memory issues, there are going to be days when your mind seems to be functioning at about half speed. You get distracted and have trouble maintaining focus, your creative thinking can't get off the starting blocks and everyone is coming up with ideas but you. The more you've relied on your quick wit and persuasive logic, the worse these days are going to be. They will derail and scare you. And if you're used to feeling like The Woman With The Perfect Mind, this has the makings of a real meltdown.

Shift gears! For starters, slow down. Don't try to overachieve if today is one of those days. Let others take the lead till you're feeling sharp again. Relax and concentrate on the other qualities you bring to every situation. Remember, your mind is not the only asset you have. Your heart is a big warm wonderful force you can use for good no matter how many things you forgot this morning.

Things to do:

1. Start writing things down or putting them in a PDA—appointments, shopping lists, task lists.

2. Make sure you have obvious places to keep things like your keys, and try to train yourself to always, always, always put them back there. Notice I said *try*.

3. Leave yourself voicemails.

4. When your brain seems to be taking a day off, catch up on your tasks and chores that don't take any brilliance. What's your favorite mindless activity? Cleaning out your purse?

5. If you're in a team situation and people are expecting you to participate, be a real team player! Let others show their brilliance today, while you take a turn in a supporting role. They'll really appreciate your backing and your cooperative attitude will remind everyone what a great person you are to have around.

6. Trust that if there is something cosmically important for you to do, the universe will make sure it happens, one way or another.

I've failed

There is always a story behind this one and the most useful thing to do is to spell it out. Write it down if possible, because you really need to get clarity on this. Without examining your thoughts and feelings here, you're never really going to get past this feeling.

Life seems to never get tired of showing us how things don't turn out the way we expect them to. When it's something that we think we have some control over, it's that much more upsetting not just to our goals, but also to our understanding of how the world works. Feeling as though you're not accomplishing what you think you're supposed to can push you into anything from a slight change in approach to a major change in your life. The thing to keep in mind is that whatever is happening, what you'll be adjusting to—if you do choose to adjust—is a closer approximation of reality. If this is a situation you plan to keep working on, put your creative hat on to help incorporate this new and better understanding of the facts.

What you're doing is successive approximation— getting closer to the truth by trial and error. It's actually how humans acquire knowledge most of the time. It's pretty rare to be right about something you've never encountered before, or to see all the details of a situation before you get into it. The fact of life is that we think we understand things, then we do the things, and as we slip, trip, and stumble our way through them, we finally come to understand them. So let yourself off the hook, for one thing. Stop thinking "failure" and start thinking "next stop on the train to wisdom city."

Things to do:

1.   Make sure you're not just comparing your life to someone else's. You are you and she is her. There is an important cosmic reason you are not her, and not living her life.

2.   How is it that you feel you're failing?

3.   On a scale of one to ten, how important is this to you, and why?

4.   Do you feel as though you let others down, or just yourself?

5.   What would the consequences be if this thing couldn't ever happen as you think it should?

6.   What alternatives would you have for reaching the same goal in a different way?

7.   Even if an action completely falls through, you still learn things from attempting it. Write those down too; add them to your personal knowledge and skills list.

My body got old since the last time I checked

Yes. It did. I'm sorry. My knees started going when I was twenty-seven. Then came the wrinkles and age spots, then my near vision gave up and took off, and when I hit fifty-five I lost my ability to digest starches and complex sugars. After that it seemed as if every year, there was some noticeable negative change as I became less fit, less strong, less flexible. Doing tai chi and kung fu several times a week was the only thing that kept me together. When I stopped doing that, my physical decline accelerated. Recently I had one skin cancer removed and now I enjoy regular pains in my knees and elbows. I'm personally not interested in taking human growth hormone, so I know that pretty much the best I can do is slow down the aging process a bit, not reverse it.

Age *and* mileage—they both start counting in these years. Both injuries and normal wear and tear have been accumulating over the years, and now they could be starting to show up and actually get in your way. You might not be ready for "low impact" and "age appropriate" yet, but if one of your activities is causing you problems, it's a good idea to make some kind of change. You do want to keep being able to do fun things for another forty years, right? The better shape you can get into now and stay in, the more fun you're going to be able to have in those years after you retire.

Things to do:

1. Show your body you love it by taking care of it. It got you this far; it deserves the right attention from you.

2. If you've ever contemplated pampering yourself, now is the perfect time to try it.

3. Balance and flexibility are as important as strength, or more so. Make sure they're on your fitness priority list.

4. Tai chi and yoga add the benefits of meditation and deep, relaxed breathing to the practice of beneficial movements. Be sure you learn from a competent instructor, and never do anything that hurts.

5. Remember—if you don't use it, you lose it. Hang onto your physical capabilities by practicing them.

6. It's always easier to keep yourself exercising if you have a buddy to do it with. Network or use the Internet or put up a notice at the gym till you find one.

7. If you do get an injury, or overexert to the point of pain and stiffness, it'll probably take longer to heal than it did when you were young. Make allowances for yourself.

Things I used to love to eat give me gas

I began to have digestive difficulties in my late forties, but it was several years later when it became a constant problem. The only thing that saved me—and the people around me—was taking supplemental enzymes with every meal. I kept hoping it was a temporary or nutritional problem, and tried to figure out what or how I needed to eat to get rid of the gas cramps and pains. Eventually I realized it was permanent. Recently I've talked to other post-menopausal women who have the same problem. One said she mixed dried apricots and prunes one morning and thought she was going to explode. She can eat apricots, or she can eat prunes, but she can't eat them together.

If I eat more than a teaspoonful of a carbohydrate food, I have to take enzymes. I carry a small bottle of them in my purse, so I'm never without them. I learned to recognize the sharp pain of a big gas bubble in my gut, and take gas pills to get rid of it. Happily I'm able to buy both products in bulk. I guess there are a lot of us out there.

It's a sad fact of life that you can't eat as you did when you were a kid because your body doesn't *need* for you to eat as you did when you were a kid. Besides having different nutritional requirements, it needs a lot less food, unless you were smart (and fortunate) enough to stay really active physically. The good result of this, though, is that you may be prompted to eat more healthily.

One interesting thing I've found is that tastes that used to literally gag me don't bother me any more. I never could eat beets when I was young, but now I love pickled beets; I'll eat them like candy. I even eat regular beets, without the extra sugar. Yes, they do give me gas, but pretty much everything gives me gas. I loved hearing that the average human passes gas fourteen times a day. Yes, I do *now*, but I never used to do that when I was young, unless I did it all in my sleep. Where did that come from? Now I can practically do it on command.

Things to do:

1.   Take notes; keep track of what you can and can't eat until you memorize it. Remember it takes twenty-four to forty-eight hours, more or less, for a meal to pass completely through an average adult gut, so when you have a problem, you can figure back how far it could have started.

2.   Some things that you can't digest after an evening meal, you may be able to handle earlier in the day.

3.   Digestive issues are just one more physical problem that can surface for the first time during menopause, robbing you of energy. If you have persistent gastric distress, work with your doctor to figure out what's causing it.

4.   Sad to say, your friends who invite you over won't know what you can't eat unless you tell them. It's embarrassing to have to admit you can't eat everything they've prepared, but it can be painful to try. Explain to them simply that you have a gastric condition that makes it impossible for you to eat that. Most likely, they'll understand.

Someone else is living the life I was supposed to

I spent years in this box, and I didn't like it at all. You're jealous of anyone who is doing work they love, or who took on a risky career and made a go of it. It took me a long time, and a lot of habit changing, to jump the hurdle from doing what I thought I was supposed to do, to doing what I wanted to do. The great thing—and maybe this is The Reason Why—was how much I learned about myself in the process.

The hardest thing I had to do was figure out what I wanted to do in the first place. That took about five years, followed by another three years of convincing myself that there was actually some way for me to make that transition. For the next three years I focused on acquiring the skills I needed to be successful at what I want, and at that point I realized I had already jumped off the Cliff of Insanity and was basically doing everything I wanted to do—a decade later!

Many women will spend long, satisfying years working at a career, only to suddenly realize in their forties or fifties that it's time to do something else. Whether you've spent years wondering what you really want to do, or you thought you knew but now it's changed, you're facing the same task—a possibly massive self-examination to find out where your new path goes.

Take as much time as you need to thoroughly examine this aspect of your life. Most of us have become conditioned to believe that we can't ever have what we want, we shouldn't expect too much, and must be willing to settle for something that keeps us alive even if it's not really what we want. You can reverse this conditioning, but it'll take a lot of effort on your part.

Things to do:

1.   When you find yourself being jealous of someone, or thinking that you want their life, spend a lot of time digging into those feelings. Do you really want to do what they're doing, or are you envious of the way they seem to have chosen their life, and are making it work?

2.   Do you know what kind or kinds of work really make you feel good? What tasks make you feel truly alive?

3.   If you have other people telling you what you should do, it's almost impossible to separate their opinions from your own. Go to your own space where you won't be disturbed, and write down what makes you happy. What makes you want to get up every day and work?

4.   Once you start to get a handle on what you really want, start writing down all the ways you've convinced yourself that it's not an option for you, or not an option at this time. These are your obstacles.

None of my so-called friends really care about me

Think about what you actually want here—what are you really asking for? To have people want to know how you feel, or what you're thinking? Or do you just need someone to pay some attention to you right now? Are you feeling an urgent need to sit down with someone over a cup of something and chat mindlessly, or do you have something you really need to talk to someone about? Maybe you just really need a hug.

You'll be more successful if you get specific. Start with your closest confidantes, and tell them what you need. Ask for their help or time. If they're not available, work your way down your list of friends and family. No help? No one home? It may be time to get out and find more friends.

Having friends in your pocket whenever you want them pretty much means having them in your hair when you don't. If you're a creative type at all, it's pretty imperative that you're able to have time alone when you need it, whether it's to work or to go get inspired. Most people don't take well to being pulled in and pushed away according to *your* needs for companionship; unless they're codependent on you, they'll have their own lives, their own moods, their own inflexibilities. What you give is probably what you're going to get. If you want to have people who stand by you, you need to be ready and available to stand by them.

A good long-term antidote for this mood is to cultivate a regular social life, doing whatever you enjoy with people who also enjoy it. It's good for you to be with them, it's good for them to be with you, and it'll be a lot easier to remind yourself when you do hit bottom, that you really do have some very nice people to call friends.

But most importantly—don't forget to be your own best friend. How much time have you spent with yourself lately? No one will ever know you as well as you do, so make sure you love yourself unconditionally and are not afraid to pay attention to what's going on inside you. Listen to your own needs. Take care of them.

Things to do:

1. Describe to yourself the ideal balance for you between time spent with friends and time to yourself. Are you getting enough of each now?

2. Say all the things you need to say, right now or as soon as possible, to yourself. Be the friend you want. Practice compassion on yourself by being compassionate of your deepest needs.

3. Done anything interesting lately? Don't neglect your mental development and emotional satisfaction.

4. Remember that the world moves on the desires of mankind. Nourish your passions and let them help you find the friendships you need.

5. If you live near a big city, the chances are really good that there are other people nearby who share your favorite interests or activities.

6. For right now, take a break and go do something you need to get done, and then feel really good about what you accomplished.

I can't believe they said that

You feel exposed and vulnerable. Or you feel hurt, betrayed, violated, manipulated, dismissed, or ridiculed. Someone who should know better, someone from whom you would never have expected such a thing, did or said something that cracked your foundation. Someone whom you count on for support let you down, or someone said something that makes it impossible to continue your life as you have been. It may have been a secret, something said in confidence, or a lie, or a truth you have no way to deal with. Or did someone you have been putting up with just finally cross a line that you can't tolerate, and you simply must respond? It doesn't matter; you have the fallout to deal with, possibly in a public way, but certainly in your personal life and how you relate to the world.

Whatever the irreversible impact that this event had on your life, the personal factor is, "Why me? Why did this person do this to me?" If you find yourself asking that question, over and over, then dig deeper. You're liable to uncover something about yourself you never realized. If they didn't intend to hurt you, or they acted without considering all the possible repercussions, then you're really better off to consider it as an impersonal act by the universe, and forget about the person who did it. Most adults speak and act without thinking on a regular basis, and it's a miracle we don't all do more harm. But that just changes the question to, "Why did the universe do this to me?"

First you have your emotions to deal with, so give yourself time to work through them all. When you're relatively calm again, do a damage assessment. What did you lose, really? Self-confidence? Part of your personal image? An ally you thought was important to you? Someone you trusted or relied on? Your job, or an important material possession? An important relationship? Our lives are made up of many things that we'd really rather not lose.

So why do bad things happen to you for no good reason? The philosophy I've developed to deal with forced change is based on the following principles:

• You can never lose anything you really need for your life.

• If you persist in ignoring signals from yourself and from the universe as to where your life is headed, Life will reach out and touch you. The size and strength of the touch will depend on what it takes to motivate you to move in your next direction.

• There are times in our lives when we think we can't change or don't need to, and this always seems to set off some alarm in the universe: "Yoo-hoo, everything is perfect just the way it is and I'm perfectly content, come give me a cosmic slap!"

You may have to be patient to get your answer as to why this thing happened to you. Sometimes the events that direct and shape our lives don't make sense until years later when we have a much wider perspective. Sometimes you'll see the same thing, in essence, happen to someone else, and the pieces will fall into place.

Things to do:

1.   There seem to be cosmic rules about being careful that everyone needs to learn. Could there have been a self-preservation lesson in this event?

2.   For the moment, while you're wondering what your options are, think of yourself as cut loose a little. What would you like your options to be? What changes would you make in your situation if you could?

3.   Did this event cause you to think about your priorities in a new light? Were you maybe not paying attention to something you've suddenly become aware of? This is your *growth of understanding*. Pat yourself on the back—you're wiser now than you used to be.

Sometimes the events that direct and shape our lives do not make sense until years later.

I'm everybody's mother

"Can you loan me some money? Can you help me with my _____? Can you drive me to _____? Can you say something to _____ for me?" Sometimes it isn't that direct. It's people lined up to tell you their troubles, complain about something in their lives—sometimes just bouncing ideas off you and sometimes dumping so much negative energy on you that you feel pounded into a pile of pulp in a hole with your name on it. Some people never outgrow their need for mothering, and you don't have to be related to them to be the one they zero in on.

On the other hand, the experience and wisdom you've acquired with age are literally strengths you provide for your family and your community. The act of passing that knowledge and understanding on to people who can and will use it is an immeasurable benefit to mankind. Who can't recall some person in their life who was kind enough to give them some insight or guidance when they needed help that made a real difference in their life? There is great satisfaction and joyful reward in being that person who can help other humans in need.

But how much is too much? Well, how much do you have time to give? The answer is, enough is whatever you say it is. You can't save everyone, or help everyone. When you don't have time or personal resources to take care of yourself, your family, and your needs, you need to say, "No." And however firmly you have to say it to have the desired effect is the right amount of firmness. No one else can tell you what your obligations are—let that come joyfully from your heart. If your intuition is telling you to cut someone off, do it with love, but do it.

Things to do:

1.   Practice saying "No." How many different ways can you decline a request for help that you don't have the time or energy to give?

2.   Always allow yourself a moment to think about it. Say, "Let me think about that for a moment." And then remember how much you have left to do today.

3.   Let your heart, not your guilt or emotions, be your guide. What's the best thing that could happen *for all concerned, including you?*

4.   You are the one who must find balance in your life. This is a life skill, and it's important for you to learn it.

5.   Remember that you might not be the best person to help in this circumstance, but simply the closest one. That's why you must follow your heart, and your intuition.

6.   Did something come up just now or recently that pulled you away from something important? Does your heart say that's okay, or is it unhappy?

No one ever listens to me

I know exactly what you mean. Nobody listens to me either. That's one of the reasons I've journaled almost every day since 1980. But even when I'm at my most invisible and least consequential, there is one very intelligent person who hangs on my every thought—me. I write about whatever is important to me at the moment, whether it's my thoughts about dark matter and the expansion of the universe, or how good the bowl of soup was that I had today at the market with my new friend. I care deeply about everything in this life, because it's the only one I have at the moment.

Sometimes we never know how we impact the world, and some days it's hard to know for sure that there actually is a reason for us to be living. If nobody appears to care what we think or say, we're missing that validation that we need in order to feel like an integrated part of our family or group. Not being heard undercuts our sense of value, and the sense that we are appreciated for all that we are.

We are all social animals and we need this reciprocation from our group—family or friends—to keep us feeling comfortable in our lives. So while this complaint may on the surface seem trivial and childish, it points to a need that is vital in us all. Every one of us deserves to be heard when we have something important to say.

When you're at one of those emotional points where you really need that acknowledgement and reciprocation from someone you care about, reach out and ask for it. If your circle of support doesn't respond, take up the slack yourself, and get whatever it is off your chest with a heart to heart with the most important person in your life—you. And make a mental note to expand your circle. Seek out new friends, and be available to listen to them when they need an ear. There's that mutual thing again.

<u>Things to do</u>

1. Write it down. You have a need to express it, so let it out right now. Then ask the universe if there is someone else who needs to know this now. But even if the answer is "No," that doesn't mean it's not important *for you*. Make a note of why it feels important.

2. It's possible that the same people who are not listening to you have a cosmic need to figure this very thing out for themselves. Think how fortunate you were to acquire this knowledge, and wish them well in their personal growth.

3. If your requests for help or expressions of needs continue to fall on deaf ears, this may be a time for you to solve your own problem. Sometimes we benefit in unforeseen ways by handling our own issues.

People are ignoring me

If they're ignoring your advice, it's probably simply because they didn't ask for it. If they're ignoring your requests, your presence, your opinions, or your constructive feedback, it's not necessarily you. It *might* be you, but it might be *them*. Think about it, and ask yourself some questions. Is it one person you think should be interacting with you more, or is it several people? Are they just ignoring you today, or has this been going on for a while? Is it all day, or just at certain times, or with respect to certain topics or situations? Exercise your mind here, do some detective work, do a little reality check before you jump to emotional conclusions.

Sometimes when your life is turbulent or even just busy, it's easy to lose track of what's going on with others. They might be really caught up in something and just don't have time to think about what might be happening with you. They might have more on their plate than they can handle right now. That doesn't mean they value you any less, or that your relationship is coming apart. And it doesn't mean that they're sick or troubled or struggling with their life, and desperately need you to intervene on their behalf.

Relationships need slack. You need to be able to move away, even disappear, and then come back. You need room to nurture yourself, to be a complex and versatile human being with many interests and a diverse circle of friends—and so does everyone else. If your steady lunch buddy cancels for a few times in a row, don't assume that it's the end. Think of your bond as a mystical band of positive energy connecting you at a higher level. Let it join you without binding either of you.

If you really get the sense that people you enjoy being with are becoming more distant, try to let go of any emotion around that. When something comes up that you'd normally share with them, then share it. Reach out as if everything were completely normal and just be the friend you want them to be. If you still don't feel you're getting the reciprocation you would like, then you're going to have to accept that, and choose what you want to do about it.

If others seem to be moving out of your life, the best option is usually to let them go with as much love as you shared with them before. Take it as an opportunity to bring someone new into your circle, someone else whom you can share and laugh and grow with. Who knows? You might find some great new lunch spots.

Things to do:

1.   Put your emotions in your pocket for a moment, and be the objective observer here. Witness the ebb and flow of interactions and relationships with others. What is really happening?

2.   It would probably be jumping to conclusions to feel that there's something wrong. It could be that you're just becoming more aware of your own needs, and more objectively aware of the actions of others. This is okay. It means you're becoming more observant.

3.   Remember that all these people around you are human beings living their own lives. Let them, so you can focus on living your life, on becoming the person you're meant to be—a strong, caring, competent individual, with your own unique destiny.

Nobody cares how I feel

This is you saying, "I _hurt_. I'm worried or scared or tired or angry or frustrated, and I need to know that I matter." Your emotions are demanding a response and if no one else is available, you need to be there and give yourself one. Express how you feel. Write it or speak it or scream it in your car, whatever will give you the release you need. You deserve that much.

It's like a timeout—for adults. You're in overload, and you as the adult supervisor need to get yourself back out of your emotions. You do that by supporting yourself, accepting where you are, and taking care of yourself while you unload whatever it is that's come up to be dealt with.

As soon as you get through the worst of the emotions, here's what you remind yourself: No one else on this planet can replace the unique and perfect being that is you. It is in fact critically important for you to be exactly where you are right now, doing exactly what you're doing. You are absolutely special, precious, and the most wonderful gift to the world that you possibly could be, in spite of how you feel at this moment.

You are the guardian and protector of all the gifts, skills and potential within you, everything you've ever learned and everything you'll learn in the future. Your mind is as extensive as the universe itself, and your body is the perfect vehicle to take you everywhere you'll ever need to go. The universe around you was shaped and evolved to be exactly what you need to reach your highest potential, a potential that is so great that you can't even imagine it at this time in your life. You are the most magical of creations, made of pure love and pure light. Embrace everything you are with a calm mind and an open heart. Accept the gratitude of the universe that you're here now, and that you're you. Love yourself unconditionally.

Things to do:

1. Stop whatever you're doing, and pay complete attention to yourself. Be your best friend, right now, and do it with all the love and care that's in you. Take yourself as soon as possible to your comfort zone, wherever and whatever that is.

2. Write, cry, talk to yourself, and express your pain, your anger or frustration. Let it out. Let it all out. You don't have to deny or belittle it, or justify it, or explain it to anyone. Just let it come out of you.

3. When you're calm, when the emotions are gone —and it might take a while—relax. Nurture yourself as you would after any great exertion. If you feel you don't understand it, write it down so you can come back to it later. It'll start making sense to you as you grow on from here.

Nobody cares what I want

Give yourself 5 points and a hug (or some chocolate) if you realize this is a trick question. This is where you need to get creative. And I mean, *get creating*. It usually doesn't matter whether anyone cares what you want, because they can't give it to you. Some will care, and some will not. The bottom line is, you're the only one who has to care, because you're the one who can make it happen. If you don't know how to give yourself the things you want and need, that's the problem you need to work on. How many things have you successfully brought into your life? Sure, you've had misses, maybe some big ones that you still don't understand, but looking back over your life, how many things that came into your life, came after you had a desire for them?

On a smaller scale, if this is about never being on the winning side of the group vote, never getting to do the things you want to do, think about expanding your personal group, or even doing some things on your own. Your desires are there for a reason—explore them. Stay safe, be practical, but pay attention to your desires. Desire is the motivating force of the universe.

Things to do:

1.   Revisit your wish list. Keep it up to date. Reprioritize it if it doesn't reflect how you're feeling. You don't have to have the biggest things on top. If you want some little thing right now, work on getting it.

2.   Take the top things and figure out some steps you could take right now to bring them into your life. If

there's something else you can come up with that's possible right now, then clarify it. Visualize it and get detailed. Note the things that aren't clear to you, and put them down as questions to think about.

3. Go over your goals in life, and tune your wish list to match it.

4. Is there anything you can do, any step you can take right now, to get closer to your goal? When the urge gets strong, take it as a hint that there *is* something you can do now. It may be something that you haven't yet thought of.

5. Read books about people who accomplish great things. Look at the problems they had to solve and look at how they approached them. Get ideas from everyone who inspires you.

6. D. I. Y.: Do It Yourself.

It's their fault

The universe has handed you a cookie you don't want to eat. What you got isn't what you asked for, it doesn't meet your expectations, and you may not have any idea what to do with what you got. You keep thinking over and over what you wanted, how clear you were about it, what a great idea it was! So what went wrong? Why in the world didn't it happen the way it should have? A–*ha*! It's THEIR fault! Everything would have been perfect if it weren't for THEM!

Other people are for the most part beyond your control. That's actually a good thing; how much of your time and energy would it take for you to manage them all? You have more or less control of yourself, and that's pretty much it. Thinking that you're really going to be able to change people so they never irritate you again is no more productive than wishing they would all be carried off by wolves.

Even when someone else seems to be causing your biggest problems, the solution to those problems is actually in you. What's happening is that the universe is presenting you with a chance to unlock some ability or strength in you that you don't know you have. That's what an obstacle is—an opportunity for you to grow yourself. Then what is a life filled with one obstacle after another? It's the path to understanding, wisdom and compassion. And of course, a lifetime business opportunity for tissue manufacturers and all makers of comfort foods.

Where are you focusing your energy right now? Is it on THEM, or is it on you? Is it on trying to get THEM to change, or on figuring out a new way for you to accomplish what you want to accomplish? Go back to your goal. Draw yourself a new picture of the situation, and make sure you include all your obstacles in that picture, including THEM. But remember— you have command of all your latent powers and abilities. However much time it takes to figure out your new solution, be sure and congratulate yourself on your new learning experience.

Things to do:

1.   Whatever the outcome of this situation, you're learning not just about life but also about you, and it's going to be knowledge that you can use for the rest of your life. It might be a little thing or a big thing, but it's part of what makes you the unique and amazing person you are.

2.   Let your challenges bring out the best in you, as well as the worst. We all have negative reactions when something or someone gets in our way, but let yourself rise to the occasion and look for a more inclusive solution.

3.   You *do* matter. This world needs you to become the whole person you are. That's why you have this opportunity, why you're you, and why you're here.

I fell down a well and I'm stuck here

Emotionally, this is like being at the bottom of a deep narrow hole with no way to climb out. Or being tied up with a cement weight chained to you. The feeling can last for minutes, or it can last for days. You might spend a lot of time here before and during early menopause. I did.

As I look back now to when I would have these spells of feeling as if I were stuck in a pit, I'm still not sure if they were more a physical issue or an emotional one. Maybe they affect all parts of our nature—mentally helpless, our hormones out of balance, tied up in negative emotions, and spiritually disconnected. The signature of this particular mode was that I always felt that I was stuck there in that pit, and could not get out.

But always after a few days of this, there would come a moment when I would realize that the whole bundle of negativity was gone, and I would be back to feeling perfectly normal. I never kept track of them, but eventually realized this was a repeating pattern. The word "pit" would come to mind, and I'd know where I was, and know that I didn't need to worry because I'd be out of it in a few days.

One of the things that occurred to me back then was that when I did find myself in one of those holes, it was because I was holding onto an idea that literally had no future. I stayed in the hole until I realized I had to let go. Sometimes I never figured out what it was that was holding me there, but I eventually developed a mantra: "I release whatever does not serve me any more, so I can go on with my life."

Things to do:

1. It'll bother you a lot less to be in this place once you begin recognizing when you're here. After all, this isn't just *any* pit—this is *your* personal pit. Own it, get to know it, and decorate it with things you love.

2. This is not a time to struggle. Practice patience and do only what calls you.

3. How would you describe how you feel? What is it like, trying to live your life when you feel this way? Put a label on it, if you can.

4. You may be really inclined to hide out during this time; allow yourself what you need to recharge your batteries. Remind yourself that this is only temporary.

5. There are a lot of interesting things you can do when you have no energy. Read a book you've been wanting to get into, watch some new or favorite movies, find things in your favorite bright colors. Give yourself a manicure. Paint your toenails.

6. It may help to have a good cry. What's your favorite "kleenex" movie?

I need some time away

Yes, you do. If you feel that way, you do. Even if it's fifteen minutes in the bathroom, or in your car. Everybody needs some time away. Not dodging anything, not hiding, but just some time where things around you are enough different to give you a mental and emotional break. Your mind may be asking you for an opportunity to think differently about something, to see it from a new perspective. You may be in an early stage of emotional overload, and your body is warning you to take a break and let off—or blow off—a little steam.

This is a time to pay attention to your senses, to your intuition. Try to arrange some time off, and go wherever you'd like to go—home to rest, to a favorite place—whatever suits the way you're feeling. See what happens. You're probably not going to be able to play hooky this way very often, but when you can, treat it as an experiment in living your highest life. Your intuition is not just there to help you take care of yourself; it's also your connection to things outside you that are of interest or value to you. Your intuition can bring you surprises that will absolutely amaze you.

Things to do:

1.   Grab your calendar and put in some time for yourself—whatever amount of time you can get.

2.   You don't have to justify this time away to anyone else. Everyone needs this, and everyone deserves it. If you feel you simply must justify it to yourself, give it a name, like Mental Health Day.

3. Don't expect that you're going to have some major revelation during this time. Don't expect anything particular at all. Just go, relax, and do whatever comes to you. Your goal is to be by yourself and enjoy it. Period.

4. If someone were to ask you, "How many different things are you involved in now?" what would you answer? How many things would you *like* to be involved in?

I have to get out of here—now

This is, "If I don't get out of here right now, I'm going to do or say something I don't want to." If this sounds like where you are, take deep, slow breaths, relax your body, and trust what you do. You will either stay or leave. Don't try to live up to some image of you, even your own. If you stay, try to feel what's in your heart and your mind. Do what makes the most sense to you. Be the calm core of yourself. Say what's in your heart; say it honestly and with respect for yourself and for the person you're speaking to. Love yourself and be there fully.

If you leave, go calmly and do what you need to do. Trust that you're doing the right thing, just as if you had stayed. Don't waste time second-guessing yourself, or beating yourself up over what happened. You've received a lesson; embrace what happened and try to understand it in the greater context of your life.

Of course, there is always the possibility of running away. Sometimes we do run away, and sometimes we just really, really want to. I was having personal issues with a coworker one time and could only think of the scenarios where I had to either speak up and say something—and I *hate* conflict —or put up with what seemed to be an intolerable situation. As I walked out of the building after work that evening, I was thinking seriously about just phoning in my resignation and looking for another job. Suddenly I had a very clear vision of an infinite string of Earths in space, one after another for as far as I could see. The message was clear to me—each Earth was a lifetime, and I could either learn how to deal with this type of problem in this lifetime, or I could come back and face it another time.

The one thing I couldn't do was run away from the problem, because the problem was part of me. It didn't take me long to decide that I might get lucky and do the right thing, and I would be off that hook forever. The next day I knew I was going to speak to that coworker, and guess what—we had a brief discussion that settled the issue, and it never came up again.

Things to do:

1.   When you're faced with an overwhelming situation, go to your center. Put your emotions in your pocket for the moment; you'll be able to take them out later and deal with them.

2.   Say or do what you genuinely feel, and if you're not sure what to do, be the calm observer and see how much you can understand of what happens. Note the full context.

3.   Think of adding positive energy to the situation, whether it's patience, compassion, balance, humor, or just your being calm and objective.

4.   If you do leave, trust that you made the right choice, and don't get sucked into the if-onlies: "If only I had stayed," or "If only I had said...." Let it go.

I can't be me here

This situation is "This place no longer allows me to be the person I want to be." If this describes your feeling—the persistent impression that where you are is not supporting you or giving you the chance to have the life you envision for yourself—it's time to acknowledge that. You may have really good reasons for staying, in which case you're going to have to figure out how to resolve this inner conflict.

This feeling is a signal to you to be working on that, getting clarity on why, when, and how you might make your exit, and on what you're going to do when you leave. Timing may not be everything, but it's definitely an unavoidable part of the puzzle. And since change is uncertainty, and uncertainty makes most people uncomfortable, you're probably going to have a lot of conflicting feelings to untangle.

Or, you might be absolutely sure of the change you're going to make, and yet not make it for years. Stay in touch with your heart. Ask yourself the tough questions, and wait till you're sure of the answers. There will always be a way to do what you have to do.

Things to do:

1.   Be as specific as you can about what part of you is not being fulfilled or empowered where you are—not because you need this to justify your choice, but to guide you in whatever change you're going to make.

2.   Whether or not to make changes in your life is up to you; you are the only one who can know if it's time for your path to go in a different direction.

3.   Go back to your core, to your core desires and your core values. Where do you want to be now, what do you want to be doing? What are the most important things in your life at this time?

4.   How will making a significant change benefit you?

5.   Have you ever had the experience of "calm knowing"? For me, that's a sensation in my body, not a thought in my head. It's a feeling of certainty that defies any questioning. How would you describe that feeling?

I want to hit something

You're frustrated or angry, and feeling it physically. If you do hit something, hit something soft; you can hurt your hand punching hard things. Pound on a sofa, your bed, or a big thick pillow. Try not to kick things unless your balance is really good and you have on sturdy shoes. Throwing physical tantrums in your middle years is a risky prospect in any case. Jumping up and down feels good, but make sure you're on level ground and not close to any large openings. We don't want to lose you.

Feeling anger doesn't make you a bad person, or say anything bad about you. Everyone feels anger. However, acting out anger physically can invite unpleasant consequences.

Regular activities that involve hitting or throwing things are great stress relievers. For some reason, doing something that makes noise seems to be more effective. Hitting golf balls at a driving range is really great, and it has a very meditative aspect because you have to relax yet stay focused.

I went to a shooting range once with a friend who showed me how to safely handle the gun, and I was absolutely amazed at how relaxed I was after an hour of shooting at targets (and consistently missing them). I think it was the repeated concussion of the gun and the noise, even with good ear protection.

Weeding and pruning also work well for me. They both relieve stress and reassert my illusion of control, and I'm destroying things I don't want in my life. If you don't have any of those options and you need release quickly, a good scream might help. Freeway screaming is great, and you can make a regular habit of it if you're a commuter.

Things to do:

1. Physical tension benefits from physical release. Treat yourself to some.

2. Keep it safe and keep it legal, but let it out. Keeping it in is bad for you, and bad for everyone else around you.

3. Keep it to yourself. Take responsibility for your emotions and release them on your own, don't let them loose on others.

4. As the emotions come out, thoughts may come out with them. Note them if you want to, they may lead you to a new understanding of the root of your anger.

5. Part of being social is learning how to deal with your emotions in a healthy way, with only positive outcomes for you and the people around you. It takes time to learn how to do this, so give yourself a little slack.

6. Take deep breaths, and release.

I just want to be left alone

Too many distractions, too many interruptions, not enough time for yourself, or just not enough space. The difference between this one and "I need some time away" may be that you're just fine being where you are and you want the other people to leave. This is a completely normal human need and one you must learn to accommodate. I can't imagine not needing some regular time alone, or not having times when you just can't handle interruptions.

Or, it may be that you're ready for more independence, more self-determination. Personal growth means personal change. As your creative drive becomes stronger, you'll need areas in your life where you'll have room to assert it. If you can't find that room in your career or your home environment, let your passions and goals guide you to places or activities where you can stretch out.

Don't assume that your life is never going to expand or change from this point. In fact, these years bring opportunities and inspirations to many, and new, even world-changing ideas to some. Open yourself to the possibility that there are new interests and experiences waiting for you. If something does come to you—a new interest, a new idea—be the nurturing mother once more. Sit on that egg—your egg—and see what it hatches into.

Things to do:

1.   When you need to be alone, make it happen. Set your boundaries and be ready to assert them, politely

and respectfully. Cut a deal, if you have to, to be with others later.

2.   If someone does not agree that you need to be alone, you can explain it if you want, but you don't need to justify it to anyone. "Because" is a plenty good enough reason. Make your needs a priority for yourself.

3.   Make appointments for yourself, dedicate that time, commit to it, and learn to say "Not now."

4.   Learn to trust your ideas as you trust your intuition. Let them show you new directions and opportunities, where you can grow new abilities and understanding. Never underestimate the power and purpose in your ideas.

I need a good cry

I used to go for days not realizing how much emotion I had backed up, then watch a heartwarming drama or a real tearjerker movie, and cry my way through a dozen tissues before I could stop. Crying and laughing are two of the best low-impact ways the body has of releasing excess emotion. I use the word "excess" because it won't even feel as if it's about anything; it's just there in you, waiting to be released. If you feel as if you need to cry, find some time and a place, and do it. Just let go.

Letting yourself cry is much healthier than trying to hold it in, block it, or push it down. Images or thoughts of people or situations may come to mind as you're crying. Let them go; don't worry about them. You're clearing out your emotional warehouse, and you don't need to hang onto any of this. You may go through phases where you cry some every day for several days, or less often for months. I remember a time when I was so tired of crying I didn't ever want to cry again, and then I cried over that. If it's interfering with your life, talk to your doctor. If it's just a colossal pain, it will eventually end. You will go back to not crying all the time.

Things to do:

1.   Relax. There's no reason you can't cry when you want to.

2.   This normally is not something you need to keep track of. You're releasing emotion. It's an effect of the changes going on inside you as your body changes, and as your mind and spirit grow.

3. If memories come up while you're crying, of hurts or distressing events in the past, let them go. It's time for you to move on from them. You don't need to force it; this is a natural process at this time in your life. Allow it to happen and let it go.

4. If something comes up as an important unresolved issue, face it from where you are now in your life. You're a powerful grownup now, not the naive and relatively powerless youth you used to be. Use your increased understanding and compassion to counsel yourself. Your goal is to understand this issue, and move on past it.

I need to go shopping

Shopping is the modern day equivalent of stalking and hunting. This is the skill of the ancient woman, the huntress-gatherer, using her intuition and experience to get there ahead of the crowds and find the important items. Or going after they've all gone, to find that one thing of value still there waiting for her.

Shopping is a vastly underrated logic- and intuition-training activity. It can also be a competitive activity, just for fun. However, it does come with a price; a bargain price sometimes, but a price nonetheless. The wise huntress only goes after what she can afford, or she learns to practice catch and release. It's just as satisfying to hold up that cashmere sweater and say, "This isn't quite the color I was looking for," then tenderly put it back where it was. Well done. And there is always next time.

There are times when your intuition will lead you to something you didn't think you need, or don't think you can afford. Listen to your intuition. Ask again if this is something you need now, or if it's something that should wait. You can always think about it for a while. Sometimes it's enough just to know that it's there. You might, in fact, be finding it for someone else. Remember, we're all connected.

Things to do:

1.   Take note of special things that happen to you when you're shopping. It's a workshop for your intuition. When you score a jackpot, congratulate yourself!

2.   Take note also, when you've wished or asked for something and your intuition leads you right to it. Give yourself bonus points if it's on sale!

3.   When you have a good sense of your stalking skills, practice them in other areas—hunting information, or contacts, or the answers to questions that take up residence in your mind.

4.   Get used to the idea that if there is a task that's important in a cosmic sense for you to accomplish, you will receive whatever things or help are required. They'll come to you when you need them.

I've lost all my sex appeal

For the last twenty or thirty years you've probably been identifying your sexuality with the way you look—attractive face, smooth skin, shiny hair, perky boobs and your girlish figure. What happens then, as those physical attributes you've grown so accustomed to seeing in the mirror begin to change?

Your greatest sex organ is your mind. If you feel sexy, you are sexy. How sexy do you want to be? Science tells us that there is no reason to think of sex as something that disappears as we get older. There's plenty of evidence that women can enjoy sex as long as they're conscious and able to feel. After that it's arguably redundant, but you're a long way from that point. If you want to feel sexy, make yourself sexy! Wear clothes and makeup that adorn you, that bring out the beauty in your features and figure. But go deeper than that; recognize within you the Eternal Feminine—your loving and nurturing nature.

For whatever reason, every form of life we know of has a masculine, or assertive aspect and a feminine, or receptive aspect—masculine energies initiate, feminine energies create. Physically, there's the fact that men make sperm and women have wombs. Mentally, there's the difference between the ability to invent or describe some new idea or thing, and the ability to bring that thing into physical existence. Both men and women have masculine and feminine abilities, but if you are a woman, the odds are that your mind and personality as well as your physical body are biased toward the side of femininity.This happy happenstance gifts you with an infinite abundance of powerful traits that you can use to make your entire world a wonderful place.

Remember your creative power, your sensitivity and intuition, your strength and resilience in the face of all manner of difficulty and opposition. Your femininity serves more than just procreation, it's the ability to hold an idea, to shelter and grow it, to nurture and guide it. At a personal level, it's the side of you that creates the home and the sense of belonging, regardless of the environment. At a spiritual level, femininity as a principle is the formative side of the Life force itself. It's the side that holds the light, or energy, of Life in every form that is manifest in our world. If you're thinking metaphysically, it's the mystery and complexity, the hidden secrets of Life itself. As a woman, that is what you embody.

Things to do:

1.   What does womanhood mean to you? Have recent events in your life expanded or diminished your ideas of what a woman is?

2.   How do your personal strengths support your idea of a complete woman? Think about all your powers to create.

3.   Set aside some time regularly to feel sexy. Celebrate your body and its marvelous and magical nature. Celebrate all the love you can feel. Embrace your whole self as a perfect expression of everything you are.

I wish I could eat all my favorite foods

Oh, yes! Don't you wish you could eat it all! All the tastes and textures and colors you've learned to love these many years. Foods that you used to scorn seem tasty and new, but that doesn't mean you've lost the desire for all those things you loved as a child. I can still taste peanut butter and jelly sandwiches although I haven't had one in years. It seems incredibly unfair that your metabolism has slowed so much that you can't eat enough to make a bunny rabbit fat. If I could lose a pound for every weight loss miracle product I've seen on TV, there wouldn't be anything left of me. If even one of them worked, it would be so great! But nope, it's the eternal diet of some sort for all those of us who don't get enough exercise to work off what we eat.

Why can't you let yourself get just that one thing? Is it because you're like me, and if you buy a package of it in the store, you'll bring it home and eat it all yourself in a day? Use your shopping skills to find a place where you can find a single serving, or if it's really rich and fattening, a single bite. Maybe you can find something healthier that has the same basic taste —for instance, applesauce and crackers replacing apple pie. If you simply *must* eat a particular food (as I must eat chocolate), then find the healthiest way—for *you*—to eat it. For me, that's bite-sized pieces of plain semi-sweet chocolate. One bite is enough to fill my mouth, and it doesn't tempt me to binge the way the sweeter taste of milk chocolate does. Also, something in most milk chocolate gives me zits. No one should have to have wrinkles *and* zits.

The thing to remember is, every time you eat something healthy and appropriate, you're doing yourself a favor. You're loving and respecting your body and your spirit. Reward yourself mentally and emotionally when you make a choice that's healthy for you—give yourself a hug, and tell yourself how smart you are. Because you *are*.

Things to do:

1.   Make a list of the things you want to eat but don't think you should. Reduce each one to its essential taste or flavor or sensation that you crave, something that if you can eat just a small amount, it'll satisfy that craving.

2.   Try to find appealing forms of healthy foods you wouldn't normally eat. If a little cheese or buttery spread or sweetener on top helps you eat it, go for it. It can help you learn to like the taste.

3.   Take control of your indulgences by scheduling small ones, every now and then.

No problem! I feel GREAT!

This age of your life is the threshold of your most creative and satisfying years. It's time to sink your roots into infinite spirit and rejoice in all your beauty and strength. You have reached your maturity, and it's time for you to take your skills and abilities and use them to nurture all the wonderful and amazing things going on in your world. Sharing yourself is the most generous gift you can give. The more you open your heart to bring out beauty and love, the more the universe will pour its beauty and love into you, and through you, out to the world.

Do what you love, and do it with everything in you. Give from your heart to everything you work on. Celebrate all the beauty in your life, all of the people and creatures and plants and things in your life that you love, that enrich your life. Give thanks for everyone who loves you.

Things to do:

1.   Celebrate everything that makes you happy. If nothing else, just say to yourself, "Whoopee, this is great!"

2.   Give love back to the things you love by taking care of them.

3.   Give voice to your appreciation for what is important to you.

4.   Embrace everything you learn about yourself, and forgive the things you want to change.

5.   Give yourself love, in every way you can.

If there's anything
that gets in the way
of loving yourself
unconditionally, let
it go.

Worksheets

This last section is a collection of worksheets you can use to explore your feelings about different aspects of your day and your life. Their purpose is to help you expand and remember the larger aspects of your life, the bigger picture, for when you get stuck in some rat hole of emotion and can't get out.

When you're feeling down for any reason, it's hard to remember what your life is like when you're feeling good. You can use these notes from better times to see yourself and your life more objectively.

An important part of keeping a balanced outlook is training your mind in the use of creative, active thinking. Creativity isn't just about being able to make things with your hands. Creativity is changing your thoughts about something you'd like to be different in your life right now, from thinking that you can't do anything to improve it to thinking that there *is* something you can do, and if you focus on it, ideas will come to you. Creativity is the act of thinking, "What can I do to make this situation better?" For example:

Negativity: "My life is so boring, I can't stand it."

Creativity: "I want to do something different and interesting. Now what is there that would be fun for a change that I can afford to do?"

Some of these worksheets you may only want to write on once, others you may want to make copies of to use whenever the occasion arises. You can save the stuff you write, as a journal, or you can write it, read it, and burn it. How much or how little you want to write is completely up to you. If anything here does not feel as though it applies to you, ignore it. If you don't see what you care about in here, create your own work sheets. Do whatever is useful to you.

I was in my mid-thirties and had recently started journaling when I began to write about the days that I felt particularly unhappy, when I would feel depressed and uncertain of where my life was going. In just a couple months I realized that I always had a couple days a month where my mood was in the dumps, to put it mildly. They came out of the blue, had no tie to anything happening at work or at home, except—guess what—they turned out to be the last two days before my period started. Surprise!

In my first year or so of journaling, besides learning to recognize my own PMS, I also found out that whenever I got a cold or mild flu, I would always feel depressed and anxious, and had a pretty much negative view on everything. It dawned on me that there was a connection between my emotions and how I felt physically. I made a decision then, to never make any major decisions when I didn't feel good.

So, what's the point in writing about where you want to be in a few years when the signs are pointing to your life being the same then as it is now? If you want something enough that it keeps coming up in your mind, you have an obligation to yourself to explore that desire and figure out why it won't go away.

For one thing, writing or even just thinking about what you want will nourish your imagination. Is there someone else you could share your stories with? Maybe your kids would like to hear them. Writing about things you love, including the things you already have in your life, is a great way to explore both the depth of your feelings and your interconnectedness with other people, places, and times. Writing about anything that means anything to you is a way to better understand those feelings, and it can also help you figure out what's really important to you at those times when you're not so sure.

A lot of the worksheets are about what makes you *you*. Whatever the meaning of your life is, it has an aspect of uniqueness that is purely centered on you and what you bring to it. Learn every gift you have, even the gifts of weakness, everything that makes you what you are. This is the hero's journey, the journey of self-discovery, the discovery of the most wonderful creation in the universe—you.

Paying attention to your own life is the only way to see what is really going on in it. You've learned about everyone else in your life; make sure you assign as much importance to yourself as you do to others. If there's anything in your life or behavior that you'd like to change, the first step to changing it is to observe it. A journal is a silent friend, and writing down your thoughts and feelings gives you the same benefits as bouncing them off another person, but minus the advice you're likely to get.

Writing is an effective way to deal with loss, and to help you let go of things that have moved out of your life. It's also a safe way of expressing emotions that you don't know what to do with. It really does get it off your chest, and you can say exactly how you feel without mincing words. That's no different from telling it to a friend. You expressed it, and now it's gone.

I like to write, so I use writing to organize my thoughts. If you're not a writer, you can still mine the worksheets for ideas to think about.

When you're down, it's hard to remember what "good" feels like. Keep notes to remind you.

#1 – Making A Menopause Journal Worksheet

A Menopause Journal Worksheet is an instant diary page you can use any time you want to record something you're feeling today, or something that happened that you'd like to delve into. With a sheet of paper, a pen, and access to a copier, you can make your own worksheet to help you keep track of feelings, issues, or physical symptoms you're experiencing. If you already keep a journal or diary, you probably won't want this worksheet unless you're a nerd like me, but if you're not used to writing down personal information about yourself, a worksheet provides a quick shortcut you can grab anytime.

There are a couple of reasons why you might want to do this. First, if you're starting to notice feelings or situations that occur repeatedly, you can gain insight into where those feelings are coming from by recording when you have them and what you think might have triggered them at this particular time.

Second, if anything about what you're feeling is bothering you in any way and you want to talk to a health professional or counselor about it, having a record of how often it happens and how much it concerns you will help them understand what you're dealing with.

To make your own menopause journal worksheet, start at the top of the page with a place to write the date, day of the week, and time, to help you see recurring patterns. Other useful things to note here are how many hours of sleep, non-sleeping rest, and recreation you've had in the last twenty-four hours. Since good sleep is the hardest thing to get during menopause, it's really beneficial for you to start noticing how much you do—or do not—get.

For recording your feelings, simply list the feelings or situations that occur in your life. You can start with the list of feelings in this book's Table of Contents, or you can write down any feelings in your own words. If "I want to throw things" is a feeling you have and recognize, use those words. Use whatever words or descriptions you want, as long as they describe what you're feeling. Then every day, at the end of the day, you can just check off whatever feelings you had, making note of any questions or insights you have about them.

If you have recurring physical symptoms that you're unsure about or just want to keep track of for a while, list those as well: hot flashes, pains, periods or spotting, any physical feeling or symptom. When you have all the items on your worksheet that you want to try keeping track of, make a few copies for later and put them where you can get to them easily. Keep one unused copy to make more from when you run out. Resist the urge to make a lot of copies at first; there's a good chance you'll want to customize it after using it a few times.

If you've never kept any kind of a journal, using any of the worksheets at the end of this book can help you think of things to write about. Any feeling on them that you recognize, for instance, might spin off into thoughts about other happenings that you feel comfortable expressing. That in turn can help you to think of your daily life in new ways.

#2 – Emergency Self–Expression

You're really upset right now and you want to do something about it.

Will it help to get some physical release first? Yell, cry, pound a pillow, go for a walk or a run. Stay safe, but let off some of that excess energy.

Go somewhere where you can be by yourself. If you're too pumped up to write, talk out loud to yourself. Say whatever comes up; get it off your chest. Be aware that you're feeling a lot of emotion right now, and whatever comes out is going to be affected by that, but say it anyway. These are your feelings and it's okay for you to let them out.

Talk about anything that happened, what your feelings are right now, and whatever you're thinking. Take deep breaths and say what's on your mind or in your heart, whatever it is. Everything you want to say is important here. Don't worry what it means or whether you should say it or not; if it wants to come out, let it.

When you calm down, or want to remember what it is you're saying, grab your journal and start writing.

#3 – Sample Journal Entry

If you'd like to try journaling for the first time and don't know where to start, here are some questions to get you going:

- How was your day today?

- What's been happening lately?

- Is there something you're happy (excited, sad, worried, frustrated) about?

- Have you had an interesting interaction with someone else?

- Are there any new things that have come into your life lately?

- Are there "people" issues you've been dealing with lately?

- Did anything funny happen that you can laugh about?

- Is there something you'd like to talk about with someone?

- How are you feeling right now—physically, mentally, emotionally, spiritually?

- Has something come up that you've never had to deal with before, and you're not sure what to do?

- Is there something coming up that you're looking forward to?

- Do you need something now—a hug? A cry? A nap? Some chocolate?

#4 – Getting To Know You

- Which of the things that you do are the most important to you?

- Have you already had experiences that have changed the way you look at life?

- What are your strongest skills and talents, both the ones you have used, and the ones you haven't gotten a chance to use?

- If you could have any job in the world, what would it be?

- If you could make any changes in your life, what would they be?

- What would you most like to accomplish in your lifetime?

- What's on your "bucket list"—what do you want to do before you kick the bucket? You don't have to explain or justify it, just write it down.

#5 – Finding Your Calm Center In The Middle Of A Situation

- Make sure you're breathing; take deep slow breaths.

- Take a few seconds to focus your attention in the center of your upper chest. Tell your whole body to relax.

- Put your emotions in your pocket for right now. You can take them out later when this is over.

- Feel the energy in your heart right now.

- Ask in your heart for the highest possible outcome for all concerned, including you.

- Say what comes from your heart honestly, respecting the others there, and with consideration for their feelings as well as your own.

#6 – Midwife Your Life

- Do you have skills you'd like to improve?

- What additional skills would you like to acquire?

- Do you have a personal growth goal, apart from skills, that you're working on now or thinking about?

- Where would you like to travel?

- Thinking ahead five years from now, what would you like to be doing? What about ten, and twenty years from now?

- Do you have secret longings?

#7 – Where Are Your Time And Energy Going?

• List the work and activities that occupy your time now.

• List any other activities that you'd like to have time for now.

• Mark the activities you'd like to scale down or eliminate.

• List any obstacles to cutting down on those activities. Are they people obstacles, commitment obstacles, or some other kind?

• How much "you" time do you have every day, or every week, or every month?

#8 – Midnight Thoughts

What keeps you awake at night? When you're lying awake in the middle of the night, what is it that goes through your mind?

Maybe it's the perfect response to that thing someone said that bugged you the whole day.

Maybe it's just some bubble of disconnected energy that makes you restless and feeling as if you need to be doing something.

Maybe it's a fear asking to be validated, a self-affirmation asking to assert itself, or your inner child asking you to stand up for her.

It may be something you have been dodging for twenty years that is no longer going to take "not now" for an answer.

It may be a worry or a feared consequence you've had buried inside you for most of your life that isn't ever going to happen and just wants you to let go of it and free up that emotional energy. You may be doing a lot of this during menopause.

If you're not sure what's on your mind, you may be able to distract yourself back to sleep with a book. Or, see if you can burp it up by walking around for a few minutes, have a bit of milk or a couple crackers, or go play your guitar or keyboard (through headphones if there are others sleeping).

Or try meditating. Sometimes deliberately quieting your mind will make it easier for the fundamental issue to present itself clearly.

If it's something clear and specific, sometimes you can buy a reprieve by acknowledging that it's present, it's urgent, and you'll take the first step toward dealing with it now—whatever that is—and finish tomorrow.

If it's bringing up anger or hurt in you, don't be surprised if you feel like crying. Grab your tissues and go for it. You'll feel a lot more relaxed after you let go.

If you have to face it now, then face it. Work through it till you feel it relaxing its hold on you. Then go back to sleep. And don't forget to catch up on the sleep you missed as soon as you can.

#9 – Your Greatest Inspirations

It's interesting to think that the oldest meaning of "inspire" is to breathe in. What if great ideas were all around us in the air, and all we had to do was take a deep breath? What if the universe held countless zillions of inspirations right now, just waiting for us to open up and receive them? What if all you had to do to get an inspiration were just to open your mind?

What are the most inspiring moments you've ever had? Write about any times in your life when you had a transcendent experience, or felt that you saw or understood something really important. What are the thoughts or images that come to you when you're feeling really connected? Do other people inspire you? Are there ways that you would like to inspire others?

You might find that ideas come to you when you see other people doing something you wish you could have done. You might get more ideas when you're in the shower, or when you're rested, or when you're frustrated. You may get great ideas about one thing, while you're working on something else.

Our culture used to write people off as contributors by the time they hit retirement age; now we know this is rubbish. People all over the country are finding new passions in their fifties and sixties, and doing amazing work. If you have unfulfilled dreams or ambitions, now is the time to go to work on them. If you're lucky enough to be alive after menopause, and the odds are that you will be, make it *your* time.

#10 – Your Deepest Satisfaction

You deserve to feel the kind of satisfaction that reminds you that life is a precious gift, one designed especially for YOU. You feel wonderful about your life; you feel deeply rewarded in the most meaningful way. These moments, rare as they are for most of us, are clues to the essence of our lives. Interestingly enough, they rarely come about unless we *do* something. What kind of something? I think it's different for everyone. It may be a very small thing, or a very large, complicated thing. But for you, it'll be special, and unique. It'll be something that gives your life meaning; something that resonates with you in a way that few other things do.

What lights you up? What makes you feel as if there is nothing in the universe as lucky as getting to be you? What were the times that made you feel that you hold a very special key to *something*?

If you're interested in having a lot more of these moments, and really get to know what they're all about, start indulging yourself by doing things you love to do. And while you're doing them, think about why you might be so affected by these activities.

When you have an occasion of deep satisfaction, celebrate it. Make a big deal with yourself about it. Ask to have more of those moments. Don't worry about how you're going to make them happen, just enjoy them, and ask for more.

Write down your request to have more experiences of deep satisfaction in your life.

#11 – All The Ways You Are A Wonderful Person

This exercise is more important than you might think. You need to acknowledge and connect with *all* the best parts of yourself. Think about all the ways that the following words apply to you. Start by picking one or two and writing down an example from your past that brings up happy memories, or one of your wishes for the future. I'll bet that if you give yourself enough time, you can remember an occasion when you embodied or expressed each one of these attributes.

- Kind-hearted
- Gifted
- Generous
- Loving
- Nurturing
- Appreciative
- Sensible
- Practical
- Decisive
- Original
- Intelligent
- Skilled
- Successful
- Protective

- Learning
- Growing
- Understanding
- Courageous
- Inventive
- Sensitive
- Passionate
- Talented
- Clever
- Insightful
- Compassionate
- Focused
- Balanced
- Shining
- Trusting
- Coordinated
- Graceful
- Gracious
- Beautiful

Feel free to add to this list!

#12 – Your Favorite Worries, Handled In A Different Way

Do you have regular worry targets in your life? Would you like to worry less and enjoy life more? If you know how to worry, then you know how to meditate. But instead of doing nothing for you except putting you in your grave sooner, which is all worry will ever do for you, meditation actually makes you feel better...which makes the people around you feel better...which makes the people around *them* feel better...and so on, and so on....

Here's how to turn a worry fest into a positive meditation. If you've never done this, it'll be easier to do it focused on a person before you try it on a situation. This will only take a couple minutes, so you can sneak this into your day whenever you find yourself being taken over by worrying. Start by selecting a person in your life whom you spend a lot of time worrying about—just one for now. Take a few moments to think of some of your favorite memories of this person, and the good feelings you have about them.

Now, holding this person in your mind, sit quietly for a moment and bring those feelings of loving affection into your heart. Concentrate on those feelings and really get into them, as if they were expanding out from your heart to fill your entire body as you breathe. As those feelings grow, see that person again in your mind, and imagine all that wonderful feeling in you flowing to them right now, just let it go and send it to them. Along with that love, send them your unconditional good wishes for everything in their life. Visualize all the love you sent and your wishes surrounding them, right now, as you relax and take deep breaths.

Once you've done this meditation a few times and you know what the steps feel like, try it on a problem or situation you've been either trying to figure out how to handle, or that you've been trying really hard to avoid entirely. Not only do you not need to have a particular outcome in mind, it's better to not think of it if you do. Just think of the situation, hold it in your mind for a moment, with all the complications and personalities involved.

Now shift your thoughts to something or someone you love, and focus on that love in your heart. Breathe into that feeling and let it grow and fill you, as much as you can in a few moments. Don't worry about how much or how little you feel the love this minute; it's your intent that matters here. Recall the situation again and let what's in your heart flow out to it, as you ask for the highest possible outcome. Focus on that for just a moment as you breathe—*the highest possible outcome for all concerned*—as you feel your energy, your love, and your good wishes flow out to that situation.

Now let go of the situation and all the parts of it and all the thoughts you have about it. Relax, keep breathing, and switch your mind to something else. It's the same as putting something in the oven. You put it together and you put it in the right place; now just leave it alone while it cooks. You've just done the best possible thing you can do to help that situation.

But let's be real—if this is one of your *favorite* worries, you are going to worry about it again. If you can't stop yourself, do the meditation again. Just like turkeys, the big ones have to cook a little longer. And you can never send too much unconditional love.

#13 – Training Your Mind To Go Higher

Ah, intuition, that inner knowing—calm, balanced, eye-opening guidance that never fears, never intimidates, never scolds. It's the silent voice, the sudden insight, the simple answer to complicated questions that pulls all the pieces together so that things at last make sense. Would you like to have that perspective, that wisdom available to you every time you have to make a choice, to help you see more clearly? To help you set aside your emotions, your fears, your worries about what the best thing really is, when others are involved?

Intuition is there; it always has been, while you've been learning how to use it, learning to trust it. It's not some other being's mind; it's your mind, your higher mind. It's part of your spiritual body that you've spent your life so far growing into. You'll always be able to recognize it because it will only give you wisdom, never anything false or self-destructive. Don't take just any b.s. for an answer; if what comes to you does not take you to a higher place, throw it out. That's not intuition.

One time I wanted to know where ideas come from, how they get in our thoughts. A day went by and I got no answer. The next day I asked more strenuously; I *really* wanted to know. That night I had a dream of being in a huge dark hall, so big that I could only see one wall, a smooth black high wall, the edges of which disappeared into the dark space around me. I walked up to the wall and saw a horizontal slit at eye level. A strip of paper appeared in the slit, and I reached up and pulled it out. I woke up from the dream. That was my answer. I interpreted it then as meaning that I could not know, or was not ready to know, how ideas come to us, just that they do.

At this point in my life, I believe they come to us in response to questions or desires. When I look back at that dream, I think I may have figured that out then, but it's taken me this long to put it into words. Perhaps a better way to say it is, they come to us in response to *doing*.

Put the universe to work for you every day. Every time you have a question, ask your higher mind, and then see what answer you get. Use that answer, or not, but remember what it was when things all work out (or when they don't). When you have a really big question, ask your higher mind. Ask whatever you want to know. If you can ask the question, you deserve to get an answer. Ask, keep asking, and be sure to be listening for the answer.

If you want to ask the question, but you're not sure you really want to know the answer, you can write it down, and say "I'm not asking this now, but I'm thinking about it." Let your mind be curious about everything. Some questions you want a secret answer to, an answer you don't think anyone you know could give you, or a bigger answer that will take the whole universe into account. Why not ask? What in the universe could you possibly *not* be supposed to know, or to understand? You're an adult. Knowing everything is part of your job.

But don't be afraid to ask little questions, either. Where is the best place to park? Should you call now or wait an hour? Should you buy this now, or will it be on sale in a week or two? Should you talk to your boss about this issue today, or should you write your frustrations in your journal, and wait and see what happens?

Once you're satisfied with the way you asked the question, let it go and wait for the answer to come. Listen calmly for the answer. It might be what you were already thinking, and it might not. It might be what you want to do, and it might not. But now you have a second opinion.

What questions would you like to get an answer to, either now or in the future?

#14 – Have An "I Give Up" Day

There is something that happens for most of us at some stage in life, usually in youth, called the Illusion of Control. You're doing the things you want to do, and you don't have to struggle much at all. This is usually a wonderful time in your life, when it's easy to feel good about yourself, others, and Life in general. You can get a lot done in that mode. Some people spend a long time there, but some see little or none of that "I'm in control" stuff after their fourth birthday. Some other people are really successful at gathering others around them who want them to be in control.

The opposite of feeling as if you're in control occurs when *nothing* goes the way you plan or the way you think it should. You never get anything that doesn't contain some compromise, you're constantly running into one problem after another, and obstacles seem to come out of nowhere just to get in your way. During this period, you may not really accomplish that much outside you, but you accomplish a whole lot on the inside. You learn to stop resisting and to become observant. You learn to stop talking, to watch and listen. You learn that other people can have great ideas too, and that's a good thing.

Until you've lived through both of these scenarios, you don't really know life. By this point you've probably experienced both, and you know them well enough to recognize when one or the other is happening, to you or to other people. You've already learned that there are times when you have to fight, and times when you have to let go.

An "I Give Up" day is an exercise in seeing what your life would be like if you were riding in the back seat, instead of driving the car. If you're tired of pushing, if you're tired of trying to arrange everything and everyone to come out right, try "I Give Up." Maybe not for a whole day, but for a few hours, or in one particularly troublesome situation.

The idea is that you're going to hand this time or this situation up to the universe to manage, just long enough for you to see what else might be possible. You don't say no; you don't abdicate any responsibilities; you just relax and do not push—and you *do not* worry. It's as if everything around you were working out perfectly, you're playing your part, but you don't have to worry about it. You say and do what's in your heart, when your heart says to, but you want to see how the universe is going to vote on it.

Take an "I Give Up" day, when you're ready, and write about how it felt.

Last Words

I'm already past sixty, and it's been five or six years since I first felt as if I had left menopause behind; actually I no longer remember exactly when it was. Half a dozen times a year or so, I have a hot flash; I had one the other day. If anything, from the other women I've talked to, I think my menopause was on the light side of average. But every feeling I list in this book, I have had. Some of them I still deal with regularly. All the ones tied to physical aging are increasing, but so are all the good things tied to spiritual growth and understanding. More and more, I'm feeling that not only were those years of menopause not a loss, but it was during that time that I really came to know myself. In those years, I began to feel that my life was really my adventure.

From perimenopause through menopause, I changed my mind about what I wanted from life about a dozen times, and yet now I can look back many years before that and see that there is a profound continuity between the choices I made decades ago and the core activities of my life now. I rewrote a lot of the rules I had for living over that time, but I can look back and see that on the inside, my essential wants and needs haven't really changed. I've been able to do an amazing number of the things I wanted to do, made some really deliberate experiments that didn't quite turn out the way I thought they would—but still, here I am, working on the things that are most important to me and still wanting to do more.

I thought of trying to share with you my new-found wisdom and understanding, but that's just me. You need to create your own wisdom, your own understanding, every moment you live and in every thing you do. Within you is your own best source. You will find every teacher and guide you need, and you will always have what you need, and do everything you have to do.

Commit your life to being your whole self, and accept nothing less. Trust what's in your heart. Trust what you do. Love yourself unconditionally, always, because you have always been, and will always be, a perfect human being.

Thank you for being YOU.

9677016R1009

Made in the USA
Charleston, SC
02 October 2011